WO 18 2 MCQ

The Ultimate Guide to Passing Surgical Clinical Finals

The Ultimate Guide to Passing Surgical Clinical Finals

MOHAMMED FAYSAL MALIK

BSc (Hons), MBBS, AICSM
FY2 Emergency Medicine, London Deanery

and

ASIYA MAULA

BSc (Hons), MBBS
CT1 Core Surgical Trainee, East Midlands Deanery

Foreword by
David E Khoo

Consultant
Upper GI and General Surgeon
Queen's Hospital, Romford

Radcliffe Publishing
Oxford • New York

Radcliffe Publishing Ltd
18 Marcham Road
Abingdon
Oxon OX14 1AA
United Kingdom

www.radcliffepublishing.com

Electronic catalogue and worldwide online ordering facility.

British Library Cataloguing in Publication Data

A catalogue record for this book is available from the British Library.

ISBN-13: 978 184619 439 9

The paper used for the text pages of this book is FSC certified. FSC (The Forest Stewardship Council) is an international network to promote responsible management of the world's forests.

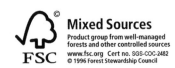

Mixed Sources
Product group from well-managed forests and other controlled sources
www.fsc.org Cert no. SGS-COC-2482
© 1996 Forest Stewardship Council

Typeset by KnowledgeWorks Global Ltd, Chennai, India
Printed and bound by TJI Digital, Padstow, Cornwall, UK

Contents

Foreword

Every patient encounter is a clinical examination: the attention to respect, the relationship with the patient, the history, the examination and above all, critical thinking, are all there. This is no more so than in the surgical examination, where the unspoken question: 'What are you going to do for this patient?' cries out from the pathology on display, begging an operation (or not, as the case may be). To pass at surgical finals as a medical student is to be awarded the right to partake in the management of a patient from a surgical perspective. So it is important to take from this the message that passing this examination is not about the supremacy of style over substance but is a true representation of the candidate's approach to the patient.

This book's approach is in the best surgical traditions of ordered thinking when it comes to the examination itself. Every system of learning requires an edifice, and this book uses that of the surgical examination to hone the thinking process. In this book, the reader will find a useful yardstick in the comparisons of the best approaches to answering a question with the worst approaches, and how best to tackle learning the subject. In reality, an inquisitive and ordered mind would do this anyway during the learning period and would therefore have no difficulty with the examination at the end. If the reader is encouraged to be thorough in learning as a result of reading this book, then the book will have achieved its purpose, not only in helping the candidate pass the examination, but in fostering the candidate's good clinical habits for the future.

By now, you should be able to tell that I have no time for the process of 'learning for the test'; I encourage you to learn the subject properly. And by the way, you will pass the exam. The experience of the finals in surgery will be more pleasant for you, and the examiner will have a more relaxing experience. The style will be the substance.

The authors of this book were among the most industrious juniors to work for me. I wondered where they would go and was delighted to hear that they have chosen surgery as a career. This book is an extension of their love of the subject and is clearly the product of much work. I admire this book and commend it to you.

David E Khoo
Consultant
Upper GI and General Surgeon
Queen's Hospital, Romford
August 2010

Preface

The key to passing surgical finals is not a secret. The ability to think logically, classify and speak coherently are all hallmarks of a good candidate. This book is aimed at teaching final-year students how to tackle the hurdle that is surgical finals. Whilst there are variations in the clinical component of surgical finals amongst medical schools, the underlying principles are the same. Having organised a successful surgical revision course during our foundation years, we have learnt many things as teachers, and this book is the culmination of our efforts.

Objective structured clinical examinations (OSCEs) have now become integrated into the postgraduate Membership of the Royal College of Surgeons (MRCS) examination, and so it is even more important that students are prepared for this examination format. Although we do not aim to teach you core surgical knowledge, we do hope that you will find the advice in this book valuable to help prepare you for the clinical component of surgical finals. The key to passing surgical finals is to do the simple things well, whilst being able to communicate in a logical and confident manner.

Well-prepared students take the initiative to create learning opportunities and propel themselves towards qualification, the necessary stepping stone to becoming a better doctor. Prepare well and you will find yourself reaping the rewards. Remember, luck has nothing to do with it.

Finally, we would like to take this opportunity to wish you all the best for your examinations.

Mohammed Faysal Malik and Asiya Maula
August 2010

About the authors

Mohammed Faysal Malik qualified from Imperial College School of Medicine in 2007. Having completed his Foundation Programme training in the North East Thames Deanery, he is due to continue on to core training in London.

Asiya Maula qualified from St Bartholomew's and the Royal London School of Medicine and Dentistry in 2007. Having completed her Foundation Programme training in the North East Thames Deanery, she is currently working as a Core Surgical Trainee in the East Midlands Deanery whilst also completing a postgraduate Masters in Medical Education.

Both authors have successfully completed their MRCS Part A examination and are currently working towards full postgraduate membership. Having published in the *British Journal of Surgery*, the authors have also had the opportunity to present at numerous meetings regionally, nationally and internationally. Their teaching record includes competitive selection during their undergraduate years as mentors for sixth-form students completing exams, the successful organisation and management of a Surgical Finals Revision Course, regular contributions to an online question bank for the MRCS Part A exam and formal training in teaching methodology and theory.

Acknowledgements

The authors would like to acknowledge the invaluable input the following specialists made in reviewing and making suggestions within their respective fields of expertise for this revision guide:

Mr Simon West FRCS (Tr & Orth)
Consultant Trauma & Orthopaedics, Northampton General Hospital

Mr Nikhil Pawa MD, LLM, MSc, MRCS
Clinical Research Fellow, Colchester Hospital University NHS Foundation Trust

Mr Saswata Banerjee MBBS, FRCS (General Surgery)
Specialist Registrar in General Surgery, London Deanery
In addition, we would like to thank the following individuals for the use of their anecdotal advice:

Mr K Marcus Reddy
Consultant Upper GI and Bariatric Surgeon, St George's Hospital, London

The authors would like to give a special thanks to the following contributors:
Muzaffar and Uzmah Qureshi, the illustrators, for their excellent line drawings.

Mr JP Greenyer for sharing his professional experience and advice with regards to the book.

Rownaq and Nabila Malik for their patient acting roles in the clinical examination skills photographs.

The medical students whom we have had the pleasure of teaching over the many years since graduating; and our mentors of particular note: Maurice A Smith, David E Khoo and Nikhil Pawa, whose guidance, advice and support during our training have been invaluable.

Finally we would like to thank Radcliffe Publishing for giving us the opportunity to publish this textbook.

List of permissions

The figures from the following books have been reproduced by kind permission of the publisher, Churchill Livingstone, © Elsevier:

Begg JD. *Accident and Emergency X-Rays Made Easy*. Churchill Livingstone; 2005.
Figure 7.19
Figure 9.22
Figure 12.4

Begg JD. *Abdominal X-Rays Made Easy*. Churchill Livingstone; 1999.
Figure 3.6
Figure 3.13
Figure 4.1
Figure 6.11
Figure 6.12

Corne J, Carrol M, Brown I, Delany D. *Chest X-Ray Made Easy*. 2nd ed. Churchill Livingstone; 1999.
Figure on page 79; Section 4.3

Jackson SA, Thomas RM. *Cross-Sectional Imaging Made Easy*. Churchill Livingstone; 2005.
Figure 2.1
Figure 2.17

The figures from the following books have been reproduced by kind permission of the publisher PasTest, © PasTest Ltd:

Wasan R, Grundy A, Beese R. *Radiology Casebook for Medical Students*. PasTest; 2000.
Figure 17
Figure 19

Visvanathan R, Feather A, Lumley JSP. *OSCEs for Medical Undergraduates, Volume 2*. PasTest; 1999.
Figure 2.27a

List of abbreviations

The following abbreviations have been used throughout this book.

A&E	accident and emergency	BRCA	breast cancer
AAA	abdominal aortic aneurysm	BTS	British Thoracic Society
ABG	arterial blood gas	CABG	coronary artery bypass graft
ABPI	ankle brachial pressure index	CAPD	continuous ambulatory peritoneal dialysis
ACL	anterior cruciate ligament	CBD	common bile duct
AD	autosomal dominant	CMV	cytomegalovirus
AF	atrial fibrillation	CNS	central nervous system
AKA	above knee amputation	CRP	C-reactive protein
ALS	advanced life support	CT	computed tomography
ALT	alanine transaminase	CVA	cerebrovascular accident
ANA	antinuclear antibodies	CVP	central venous pressure
AP	anteroposterior	CX	cross match
APTT	activate partial thromboplastin time	CXR	chest X-ray
ARDS	adult respiratory distress syndrome	DIPJ	distal interphalangeal joint
ASIS	anterior superior iliac spine	DMARD	disease modifying anti-rheumatic drug
ATLS	advanced trauma life support	DoH	Department of Health
AvF	arteriovenous fistula	DRE	digital rectal exam
AXR	abdominal X-ray	DSA	digital subtraction angiogram
BCC	basal cell carcinoma	DVT	deep vein thrombosis
BKA	below knee amputation	EBV	Epstein Barr virus
BM	Boehringer Mannheim	ECF	extracellular fluid
BOO	bladder outflow obstruction	ECG	electrocardiogram
BP	blood pressure	EMG	electromyogram
BPH	benign prostatic hyperplasia	ENT	ears, nose and throat

ERCP	endoscopic retrograde cholangiopancreatogram	JVP	jugular venous pressure
ESR	erythrocyte sedimentation rate	KUB	kidney, ureters, bladder
EUA	examination under anaesthesia	LDH	lactate dehydrogenase
EWTD	European Working Time Directive	LIF	left iliac fossa
FAST	focussed assessment sonogram in trauma	LOS	lower oesophageal sphincter
FBC	full blood count	LFT	liver function test
FDP	flexor digitorum profundus	LUTS	lower urinary tract symptoms
FNAC	fine-needle aspiration cytology	MC&S	microscopy, culture and sensitivity
FOB	faecal occult blood	MCPJ	metacarpo-phalangeal joint
FY1	foundation year 1	MDT	multidisciplinary team
G&S	group and save	MI	myocardial infarction
GCS	Glasgow Coma Scale	MRCS	Membership of the Royal College of Surgeons
GGT	gamma glutamyl transpeptidase	MSU	mid-stream urine
GI	gastrointestinal	MT	metatarsal
GMC	General Medical Council	MTPJ	metatarsal-phalangeal joint
GP	general practitioner	Na	sodium
GTN	glyceryl trinitrate	NBM	nil by mouth
Hb	haemoglobin	NG	nasogastric
HDU	high dependency unit	NHS	National Health Service
HIV	human immunodeficiency virus	NICE	National Institute for Clinical Excellence
HR	heart rate	NMSC	non-melanoma skin cancer
HRT	hormone replacement therapy	NOF	neck of femur
IBD	inflammatory bowel disease	NSAID	non-steroidal anti-inflammatory drug
INR	international normalised ratio	OA	osteoarthritis
IPJ	interphalangeal joint	OCP	oral contraceptive pill
ITU	intensive treatment unit	OGD	oesophago-gastro-duodenoscopy
IV	intravenous	ORIF	open reduction internal fixation
IVC	inferior vena cava	OSCE	objective structured clinical examination
IVU	intravenous urogram	OT	occupational therapist

PA	posteroanterior	SIRS	systemic inflammatory response syndrome
PCA	patient-controlled analgesia	SLE	systemic lupus erythematosus
PCL	posterior cruciate ligament	STI	sexually transmitted infection
PCKD	polycystic kidney disease	TB	tuberculosis
PE	pulmonary embolus	TCC	transitional cell carcinoma
PIPJ	proximal interphalangeal joint	TED	thromboembolic deterrents
PPI	proton pump inhibitor	TFT	thyroid function tests
PR	per rectal	TIA	transient ischaemic attack
PAD	peripheral arterial disease	USS	ultrasound scan
SBP	systolic blood pressure	UTI	urinary tract infection
SCC	squamous cell carcinoma	UV	ultraviolet
SFJ	saphenofemoral junction	VUJ	vesico-ureteric junction
SEPJ	subfascial endoscopic perforator surgery		

To my best friend … for always believing in me.

MFM & AM

I would like to thank my parents, particularly my mother, without whose guidance and support I would not be the doctor that I am today, and my brother, Ashfaq, for making it all worthwhile.

MFM

I would also like to thank all my family, particularly my brothers, Shakeel and Tanveer, and my sister, Uzmah, for their enthusiastic support and encouragement through all my endeavours, my mother for helping me to become the person I am today, and finally my husband for being my pillar of support.

AM

CHAPTER 1

Introduction to surgical finals

1.1 INTRODUCTION

Surgical teaching is often poorly structured in medical schools, where an emphasis is placed on medical finals, and surgical finals only seem to get a brief mention in the last few weeks leading up to the examination. Learning whilst on surgical attachments is ad hoc at best, often with very little time dedicated to teaching you the large number of history taking, examination and practical skills required. This is primarily because the great majority of surgical knowledge and technique is learnt by doing; it is an apprenticeship by its very nature. However, this does not mean you must spend endless hours in the operating theatre hoping for someone to teach you anatomy. This is a pointless exercise in a time when finals are looming. You must use your time efficiently and effectively by concentrating on what you need to know to pass the exam.

We often find the candidates who seem to know the most struggle during clinical examinations, whereas their colleagues who may not know as much are doing better. Their successful technique is no secret. The aim of this book is simple: to teach you how to think logically and communicate in a thoughtful but structured manner. This will enable you to not only demonstrate your breadth of knowledge but also your depth of knowledge.

It is necessary to pause here and emphasise this fundamental point to you: it is your breadth of knowledge that the examiner is interested in. There is no point in knowing the pathophysiology of digital clubbing when you cannot name the causes. We aim to teach you the basics and hopefully enable you to know these well, because it is this that scores you the marks and helps you to pass finals.

Students often ask us what key skills they need to pass surgical finals. While there are many skills that make a good surgeon, for purposes of finals the most important factor is knowing your basic core knowledge inside out as well as any relevant anatomy; you must also be able to think and speak like a surgeon. We emphasise these key skills throughout this revision guide, repeating ourselves as needed because we know it scores you marks and helps you to achieve your aims.

While the majority of topics we cover will be the basics, we will endeavour whenever possible throughout this book to demonstrate to you what constitutes an honours response compared to an average response to a viva question. In cases where we have described this, the honours response is in addition to what the average or good candidate had stated earlier, so you should aim to learn both responses. Furthermore, we have highlighted questions or cases that are considered difficult or at honours level. And unless otherwise stated, the answers we provide to such cases will be at honours level. This way we hope that you can identify what is needed to score the top marks in surgical finals.

Wherever possible we describe to you exactly what you should say in the examination, as if we were in the examination with you. These descriptions are given in italics and take the first-person perspective.

Ultimately, our objective is to teach you to be a confident and competent candidate so that you can pass surgical finals comfortably.

1.1.1 Common reasons for examination failure

For those of you reading this and thinking that there is no way you will make the same mistakes we have highlighted throughout this book and feel that this is all common sense, take a step back and a moment to think of your predecessors who were in the very same situation and felt the exact same way before their examination. It was they who unknowingly made these mistakes. That is the paradox here; common sense goes out of the window when you are stressed, especially with the idea reverberating around in your head that five years of hard work may be thrown away in one swift afternoon. Fear is powerful, but it can be a powerful motivator too; use it to your advantage. One of our surgical mentors in the build-up to finals once likened surgical finals to a war, where we are the soldiers, and the weapons we have at our disposal are our examination skills, our logical thought processes, coherent communication skills and lastly our knowledge of anatomy. The examination itself was of course the enemy, but equipped with our skills and training we could defeat this enemy in style and with our heads held high. We remember one candidate even saying that he quite enjoyed finals and the rush of the battle. Needless to say, if you prepare for finals with this in mind, you will find that you will be at an advantage and will hopefully be successful.

Final examinations are not easy. Do not listen to your senior colleagues who say they are, as we mistakenly did. They are only speaking in hindsight. While it is true that the purpose of finals is to pass as many of you as possible, as opposed to postgraduate exams where the purpose is to pass as few as possible; the pressure of passing finals and becoming qualified doctors, coupled with the pressure of being matched to a likeable job, makes finals an-all-or nothing event. Hence, the most important piece of advice we will give you is to prepare well, or you may find yourself on the losing end.

Poor communication

When students are asked a question they are unfamiliar with, they tend to display what is affectionately known as the 'gold fish' sign. That is, they stand in front of the examiner with their mouths opening intermittently, trying to speak, but with no words coming out. You cannot score any marks if you say nothing. This is a shame, as most examiners want you to pass and are often urging you to say something – anything that may score you points.

For those who do manage to speak, they often demonstrate what is colloquially known as 'knight's move thinking', where they tend to talk on an unrelated topic and then randomly change to a completely different train of thought, almost as if plucking answers out of the sky. This is the classical case of a student who does not classify or structure his or her answers.

Surgeons love their definitions, and not knowing a common surgical definition does not hold you in good stead. Do not make up definitions; be aware of the common ones and know them well.

Candidates who are ill-prepared for finals have underestimated the level of anatomy that is required. While you would not be expected to know detailed anatomy, it does not look particularly reassuring to an examiner when a candidate points to their respective groin when trying to describe the borders of the inguinal canal; what we like to call the 'pointing sign'. You must be able to describe anatomy using correct anatomical terms as you would do during a telephone conversation. Some students like to place their hands behind their backs so as to avoid the temptation to demonstrate to the examiner their own inguinal canal anatomy. In the stress of the examination, we have seen candidates do all sorts of things; do not let the pressure of the situation get the better of you.

Poor examination skills

There is no excuse for a candidate to attend finals, having never examined an abdomen or hip before. There are ample opportunities in the wards and clinics. You must be competent in your examination technique and slick in its execution. While there are acceptable variations in technique, a poor clinical examination will make you lose many marks.

Behavioural issues

Believe it or not, in the past, candidates have argued with the examiners, and no doubt some candidates will continue to do so in the future. When an examiner says that you are wrong, even if you know that you are right, just accept the examiner's will. It is far better to move on to a new topic and score points than to argue your case. The examiner will almost certainly not accept that you are right and will certainly not admit to you that you are. You do not have the time, and in either situation the only person who will suffer is yourself.

Do not be rude or make haste with any actors, they too are scoring you, and it may well be that their aggregate scores are the decisive ones. Under any circumstances, do not hurt or cause pain to the patient. In some medical schools, this results in an automatic fail. Remember that although this is an examination and the patients are likely to be actors, this does not excuse you from such behaviour, as you will be a working professional soon; the examiners want to see that you will be a caring and empathic doctor. Do what you would do in actual clinical practise. If you know something may hurt the patient, then mention this to them before you do it. Little things like this go a long way to build rapport with a patient and score you most of the communication skills marks that are available; we assure you there are many.

1.1.2 Revision techniques

Given that many medical school curricula pay very little attention to surgical teaching, we suggest you set up a tutorial group with several of your friends and recruit a general surgery registrar to act as your tutor at one of the local teaching hospitals. The registrar can then take you around the wards and show you the sort of cases you are likely to come across in finals. If you are really lucky, your tutor may even be the one set the task of recruiting patients for finals, and you will have an insider's advantage. If you do not know a surgical registrar, then the next best place to look is the postgraduate teaching centre, which often keeps a list of doctors who are keen to teach and will help you to contact them.

We find that the best way to learn surgery for finals is to focus your learning objectives and practise. The tutorial group will help facilitate this. Your tutors are ideally placed to assess your examination skills, critique your presentation skills and push your knowledge to the limit in the viva. You are essentially having a mock OSCE, with the benefit of receiving immediate feedback. Also, you will learn from the mistakes of your colleagues, and you will pick up on things they did well so you can incorporate this into your routine. Never underestimate the power of group learning. Perhaps, your percussion technique is inadequate and only by watching your colleagues would you have identified this, thus helping you to focus your learning needs.

With finals, we sometimes find students locking themselves away in their rooms. This is the wrong approach; there is power in numbers. The tutorial group gives you the opportunity to liaise with your colleagues who are in the very same situation as you. You may find that your colleagues have been given hints and advice on what is likely to come up in the exam; they can be a useful resource.

We suggest you start early, ideally several months before finals, and decide on the topics you wish to cover with your tutors; remember they are in full-time employment in a busy speciality, so you need to give them adequate notice. For the more specialist areas, such as vascular or orthopaedics, it is probably best to recruit a registrar from those specialities separately.

We cannot emphasise the benefits of a tutorial group enough; this is how we prepared for finals and it was invaluable. You have the safety net of being able to examine poorly in front of your tutors, ask silly questions and be corrected, rather than make those same mistakes in finals itself.

If time does not permit this or you are unable to set up a tutorial group, practise as often as you can until it's engrained into your mind and becomes second nature. Practise with your friends, family or even by yourself using pillows or having a viva discussion with yourself in the mirror; it doesn't matter so long as you practise. It is all too easy to crumble under the pressure and anxiety of finals, but with repetition and continual practise you will find yourself in auto-pilot mode and will fly through the actual examination.

1.1.3 The examination itself

Clinical surgery finals will be unlike any other examination you have taken. However, most students could probably predict the likely cases that are to come up in the examination itself; we have already done this for you.

The majority of marks in surgical examination stations are from inspection alone, so you must say what you see. The examiner will not know that you have noticed the bilateral leg amputation unless you have said so; do not assume anything.

Do not rush when talking to the examiner, classify your answers as we will describe throughout this revision guide and do not under any circumstances argue with an examiner, make jokes or be rude. This is an exam – treat it as such.

Examiner's Anecdote

'I could not believe he had the nerve to say I was wrong. I am the examiner, I am marking your examination, and do you really want to argue with me?'

Some medical schools insist you wear your short white coat, whilst others are not so strict on the precise dress code in the examination, as long as it is smart and conservative. The examination is not a fashion show, but certainly do not wear jeans, as this is unprofessional and simply not acceptable. For women, in particular, it is important that you do not wear low-cut tops or too short a dress or skirt. Firstly, you do not want to be uncomfortable during your examination by constantly having to adjust your clothes. Secondly, it is unprofessional. While you are unlikely to be negatively marked for your attire, first impressions do count for a lot. So keep it simple and professional.

Examiner's Anecdote

'He wore bright pearly white crocodile shoes! I couldn't keep my eyes off his white shoes; they were so bright it was distracting'.

And finally, sometimes it's okay to have no idea what to do, as long as you're confident in your answer. Think logically, demonstrating your breadth and depth of knowledge, and you can convince the examiner that you actually do know the answer. We hope that by the end of this book, this will be the case. Good luck.

1.2 SURGICAL TALK

Surgeons tend to talk in a very similar fashion to one another, as this helps communicate information succinctly and efficiently. Having a clear structure in your mind when approaching any question a surgeon is likely to ask you will hopefully enable you to remain calm when asked bewildering questions and help you to come out with a logical and intelligent answer, even if you haven't actually answered the question. Even if you do not know the answer you can give the impression to the examiner that you do know. This will be evident from the way you answer the question, rather than what you say. This is the reason why the well-known surgical sieves are widely used.

1.2.1 Eponymous names, rules and signs

For every generic name to an instrument, scar or anatomical structure, there is always an eponymously named one. And sure enough the surgeon will know this. Compared to medicine, where eponymous names are being phased out, surgery tends to retain their use. It is therefore important that you are aware of the common eponymous names or signs. They may well be asked in your viva.

When one of the authors was doing finals, he was asked to name a renal transplant scar, to which he responded using the correct anatomical description. He was told to tell the examiner the eponymous name or the 'proper name', as the consultant surgeon exclaimed. So, do not underestimate the power of knowing these little facts. The scar is eponymously named the Rutherford Morrison scar.

Perhaps, the most famous eponymously named law you will come across is Courvoisier's Law, which states: 'In the presence of jaundice, if there is a palpable gall-bladder in the right upper quadrant, then this is unlikely to be due to stones'. This therefore suggests that the cause is likely to be a cancer or any other cause aside from gallstone disease.

Definitions

Surgeons love definitions, and unsurprisingly there is very little variation in the defini-tions that are used, so long as you include certain key words. For example, when asked what an aneurysm is, you can either reply by saying:

'A dilated blood vessel'

(Average Response)

'This is the abnormal dilatation of an artery to more than 1.5 times its original parent diameter'

(Good Response)

'This is the pathological, localised, permanent dilatation of an artery to more than 1.5 times its original diameter involving all three layers of its parent wall'

(Honours Response)

You can see the difference in the responses given. The better responses clearly dem-onstrate the understanding of an aneurysm's pathophysiology and its differentiating features from other similar anatomical structures such as a pseudoaneurysm, which is a common differential. This is where the dilatation does not involve all three layers of the wall and is essentially a haematoma around a damaged blood vessel that commu-nicates with the vessel lumen. The three layers from deep to superficial are the tunica intima, media and adventitia. The average response is inadequate, as a dilated blood vessel could also be an ectatic artery, so it is important to state the degree of dilatation, because the dilatation may not be classified as being aneurysmal. Ectasia is when the dilatation is only mild.

Discussing aetiology

In the stress of the examination, it is easy to try and list as many causes of a condition as quickly as possible. However, this is the wrong approach, as you are only demonstrating your ability to memorise lists; a list that you will no doubt soon forget.

Authors' Anecdote

'He regurgitated five differentials before I even finished my question! He then sat back and thought he had done enough to pass! I told him I was impressed by his memorisation skills. It is far better for you to classify your answers and state them clearly and confidently then to reel off a list you clearly memorised the night before'.

It is much better to classify or structure your answers using well-accepted surgical sieves. In our experience, we find that surgical sieves you have constructed yourself are the ones you tend to remember the best.

In general, if you are ever asked about the causes of a disease process involving a hollow viscus, it is best to classify your answer with regards to how the disease process mechanically affects the lumen, the wall and outside the wall of that parent structure. For example, if you are asked for the causes of bowel obstruction, you may answer:

'The most common causes of bowel obstruction in general in this country are postoperative adhesions followed by hernias and cancers'.

(Average Response)

In addition to the above:
'Small bowel obstruction is more common than large bowel. The most common causes of small bowel obstruction are adhesions, hernias and cancers. The most common causes for large bowel obstruction are cancers, diverticular disease or a volvulus'.

(Good Response)

In addition to the above:
'However, there are many causes of bowel obstruction; they can be divided into mechanical and non-mechanical causes. Mechanical causes can be classified according to their relation to the bowel wall as in the lumen (luminal), in the wall, or outside the wall (extramural):

Table 1.1: Mechanical causes

Location	Pathology
Luminal	Gallstones, meconium, intussusception, impacted faeces, worms, foreign bodies, etc.
Extramural	Adhesion, cancers, hernia, volvulus.
In the wall	Congenital stenosis, strictures, inflammatory bowel disease, diverticulitis, cancer, radiation colitis.

Non-mechanical causes, also known as a paralytic ileus, are due to postoperative abdominal surgery, mesenteric ischaemia and metabolic causes such as hypokalaemia, uraemia, hyperglycaemia and hypothyroidism'.

(Honours Response)

Another common aetiological sieve is where the causes are classified into their originating physiological system. This can be demonstrated when, for example, you are asked the causes of digital clubbing:

'The causes of clubbing are idiopathic, lung cancer, inflammatory bowel disease and cystic fibrosis'

(Average Response)

The most common cause of digital clubbing is idiopathic. However, there are many causes of clubbing, and they can be classified into:

Table 1.2: Causes of clubbing

Classification	Causes
Gastrointestinal causes	Inflammatory bowel disease, primary biliary cirrhosis, celiac disease.
Respiratory causes	Bronchogenic carcinoma, suppurative lung disease (e.g. bronchiectasis), cystic fibrosis, mesothelioma, fibrosing alveolitis.
Cardiac causes	Congenital cyanotic heart disease, endocarditis.
Other causes	Familial, idiopathic, Graves' disease.

(Good Response)

While the average response is acceptable and will score you some points, the subsequent response demonstrates the breadth of knowledge required to excel in finals.

Discussing investigations

When you discuss investigations, it is helpful to classify them. This helps you to not only order your investigations in a logical manner but also to remember what the next most appropriate investigation is. Remember, always move from simple or non-invasive to invasive and reserve specialist investigations until the end, once all the basic ones have been done. Below, we describe an example using the acute abdomen as a case:

Investigations can be divided into simple bedside tests, blood tests and imaging:

Table 1.3: Investigations

Investigations	Tests
Simple bedside tests	**ECG:** To rule out cardiac ischemia or MI as a cause. **Urinanalysis:** Useful to look for blood if you are considering renal calculi, a UTI or to perform a pregnancy test in a woman. **BM:** To check for the blood sugar level, especially in suspected cases of diabetes presenting as abdominal pain.
Blood tests	*Simple tests:* **FBC:** To check for a raised WCC in infection or anaemia if GI bleed. **U&E:** To look for dehydration, renal failure, raised urea in cases of an acute gastrointestinal bleed, or electrolyte imbalance secondary to massive fluid shifts in pancreatitis or cases of bowel obstruction. **LFT:** If you suspect acute cholecystitis or to look for an obstructive jaundice **Amylase:** This is compulsory in cases of an acute abdomen; it is raised in acute pancreatitis to at least greater than three times the upper limit of normal. **G&S:** If you expect that the patient will need an operation or if there is any blood loss, then it is useful to send a sample to the laboratory. **Cross match (CX):** If you expect that the patient will need an operation and will require a blood transfusion, you can cross match now, e.g. an upper GI bleed that is being taken to theatre. **ABG:** If your patient is particularly sick, this will help to gauge how unwell the patient is; the lactate and pH are helpful indicators of the level of shock and can help unmask conditions such as mesenteric ischaemia. **Specialist tests:** This depends on the diagnosis.

Table 1.3: Investigations (*Continued*)

Investigations	Tests
Imaging	***Plain films*** **Erect CXR:** If you suspect a perforated intra-abdominal viscus you will be looking for air under the diaphragm. The film is taken with the patient sitting upright for at least 20 mins prior to the film being taken, as the air will need time to rise and demonstrate a pneumoperitoneum. Be aware however that this sign is only present in up to 80% of cases. **AXR:** If you believe the patient may have bowel obstruction. **Contrast films:** This depends on the case but can include a gastrograffin enema if you are thinking of bowel obstruction or an IVU for ureteric colic. ***Ultrasound*** **USS liver:** To scan the biliary tree for evidence of gallstones or to measure the size of the common bile duct in suspected obstructive jaundice. ***CT scans*** **CT KUB:** This is now the first-line investigation for renal calculi **CT abdomen/pelvis:** This depends on the case but is useful in patients not responding to treatment and in whom urgent surgical exploration is not mandated.

You may choose to add additional blood tests or other specialist tests depending on your diagnosis. In the case of pancreatitis, for example, you may wish to do several tests that help score the severity of the attack, such as requesting a blood glucose, calcium levels, liver transaminases and a C-reactive protein.

Discussing management

Whenever a surgeon asks you to discuss the management of a condition, the word management here does not solely refer to treatment. It typically covers the entire clinical encounter, starting from the history, the examination, investigations, your list of differentials and finally the treatment options available. So when you structure your answer, ensure you state this. Usually the examiner will ask you to skip to the treatment options, in which case you should structure your answer as follows.

Treatment options can be either: conservative, medical or surgical.

Table 1.4: Treatment options

Treatment	Options
Conservative	This generally includes anything non-surgical. This may be in the form of IV fluids, NG tube for drainage of stomach contents and urinary catheterisation.
Medical	This includes any drugs that may be given, e.g. analgesia, antibiotics, etc. This may also take the form of more invasive but non-surgical treatment options, such as injection sclerotherapy in varicose veins or injecting haemorrhoids. Some surgeons would argue that endoscopic treatment options fall under this category.
Surgical	This is any surgical procedure performed to treat the condition.

There is a special note on discussing chronic debilitating conditions such as osteoarthritis or cancers. This always takes a multidisciplinary team management approach with input from various disciplines, including occupational therapists, physiotherapists and clinical nurse specialists. Ensure you put this across in your answer.

Examiner's Anecdote

'When he mentioned an MDT approach to treating arthritis with input from the OT and GP, I almost jumped out of my seat! That was impressive; clearly he knows what happens in actual clinical practise'.

Discussing surgical complications

Whenever you discuss postoperative complications, it is best to structure your answer into two main categories: complications arising due to surgery and those from the anaesthetic. There are many anaesthetic complications, and it is unlikely that you will be asked about them in finals. For surgery, however, the complications can be further divided into complications that arise specific to the surgical procedure in question or in general being related to any surgical operation. Furthermore, the specific complications can then be divided into their likelihood of occurrence in terms of postoperative time, by which we mean immediate, early and late complications.

So you can see that even by the time you get onto specific postoperative complications you would have been talking to the examiner for at least a minute. You would have demonstrated that you are aware that there are many postoperative complications, not necessarily from the operation itself. For example, it is easy to mention one or two well-known complications of an inguinal hernia repair, but this does not show your breadth of knowledge.

We will demonstrate this approach using postoperative thyroidectomy as an example.

Viva questions

Q1   This 25-year-old woman has just had a total thyroidectomy for thyroid cancer. What are the possible postoperative complications?
- Complications can arise secondary to the surgery itself or from the anaesthetic.
- Surgical complications can be further divided into complications that arise specific to thyroidectomy or general to any surgical operation.
- Complications specific to thyroidectomy can then be divided into their occurrence in terms of postoperative time, into immediate, early and late complications.

Postoperative time is a generally well-accepted timeline of events. Immediate events occur within the first day of the surgery and include the operation itself, although it is safest to say 'intraoperatively' if you want to emphasise a complication that occurred when the procedure was taking place. Early usually denotes the period after the first day up to several weeks postoperatively. Late complications tend to occur many weeks after the procedure and denote any complications occurring in a time 3 weeks after the original procedure.

Table 1.5: Postoperative complications

Postoperative time	Complications
Immediate **<24 hrs**	Primary haemorrhage, laryngeal oedema, thyroid storm, damage to the surrounding structures including the trachea and laryngeal nerve.
Early **<3 weeks**	Reactionary haemorrhage, hypocalcaemia (from inadvertent removal of parathyroid glands), infection.
Late >3 weeks	Hypothyroidism, keloid scar formation, recurrence.

Primary haemorrhage is any blood loss that occurs at the time of the operation; secondary or reactionary haemorrhage typically occurs secondary to a rise in BP. Haemorrhage or laryngeal oedema compromising the airway is a surgical emergency that should be managed according to basic airway management principles (*see* Chapter 8, Principles of surgical emergencies). Most importantly, the surgical clips should be removed to facilitate evacuation and help relieve the immediate airway compromise, which buys time before definitive surgical evacuation is possible. That is why surgical clip removers are always by the bedside of post-thyroidectomy patients; watch for this next time when you visit the ENT ward.

1.3 PRINCIPLES OF A CLINICAL ENCOUNTER

With any clinical encounter, whether it is an examination station or a test of clinical skills, the same general principles apply. There are marks available for beginning and ending a clinical encounter appropriately. Below we describe the key points you will need to remember.

The clinical encounter

Introduction
✔ **Wash your hands**
- There will be alcohol gel available at each OSCE station to wash your hands; this must be done at the beginning and end of every station.
- Almost all medical schools award marks for doing this.
- NICE have also issued guidelines specifically stating that washing of hands is mandatory.

Authors' Top Tip

It is not enough to say that you will wash your hands, you must actually wash your hands to score the points!

✔ **Introduce yourself**
- You must introduce yourself using your full name and current medical student status.
- Use the patient's name if offered, or clarify his or her name at the beginning.
- Always be polite and courteous, and use the patient's surname.

✔ **Explain purpose, gain consent and ask for a chaperone**
  - As with any clinical encounter, you must gain consent first by explaining the purpose of the examination and check whether the patient agrees for you to continue.
  - This is especially important for intimate examinations where you must turn to the examiner and specifically ask for a chaperone.

✔ **Expose patient adequately**
  - This clearly depends on the situation, but in general you should ask the patient to expose as much as possible whilst maintaining your field of vision and preserving his or her dignity.
  - If you are conducting an intimate examination, you must allow the patient privacy to change.
  - More often than not, the patient is already adequately exposed.

✔ **Position patient appropriately**
  - This is particularly important in the clinical examination stations, where correct patient positioning will help make your examination easier.
  - E.g. asking the patient to sit on a chair while you examine the thyroid gland.

✔ **Build rapport**
  - There are often numerous marks available for building a good rapport with the patient. Informing the patient of what you are doing as you go along helps to alleviate anxieties as well as reminds you of the examination routine that you have rehearsed many times before.
  - This is of utmost importance when conducting intimate examinations, as there may be intrusive parts to the examination that may be uncomfortable for the patient, and by explaining and discussing this beforehand with the patient they will know exactly what to expect and this will help make them feel more comfortable.
  - If you need the patient to do special manoeuvres, use short and succinct instructions, as you do not want to confuse them; alternatively you could demonstrate to them what it is you want them to do.
  - Finally, always ask about pain and avoid starting with that part of the body if at all possible. If you know that your examination may exacerbate any underlying pain, take the time to explain to the patient that your examination may be slightly uncomfortable but should not be painful. Assure them that if you do cause pain you will stop.

Authors' Top Tip

Remember, most medical schools will fail you if you cause the patient pain, so be gentle and warn the patient beforehand.

Complete the encounter

✔ Thank the patient
  - Always thank the patient, and if undressed ensure that the patient is comfortable and is able to redress.

- If there is a blanket, then offer it to him or her.
- If you have just finished an intimate examination, you must again give privacy to redress.

✔ **Wash your hands** (the second time during the station)
- You must actually do this; do not simply offer to do so. We emphasise this point, as some medical schools negatively mark you if you do not wash your hands again; you have been warned.

✔ **Further examination**
- On the whole, use this opportunity for examinations that you feel are necessary but time does not permit.
- A typical example would be conducting a DRE after completing an abdominal examination.

Examiner's Anecdote

'When asked if the candidate would consider performing a digital rectal examination as part of his abdominal examination, the reply was "that is only written in the books!" and the expression on his face was that clearly it was an unacceptable procedure. You must say even if it is not practical to perform in the examination setting that you would want to perform a DRE'.

- However, do not be lazy and take this as an opportunity to simply state you would do something that you could have done in the OSCE station.
- This is particularly true when you need to examine both sides of the patient in a hernia exam; it is best to actually start examining the opposite side, as usually the examiner will be happy to see that you have considered this and will stop you once they are satisfied that you understand the importance of demonstrating the presence or absence of a hernia on the opposite side.

✔ **Present your findings**
- You must turn and face the examiner, then summarise your findings whilst maintaining eye contact as you find comfortable.

Authors' Top Tip

Do not fidget with your hands or look back at the patient; some students like to fold their hands in front or behind them in an attempt to seem professional; do whatever makes you comfortable and be confident in your approach.

1.4   COMMUNICATION SKILLS

1.4.1   Obtaining consent

Some medical students may argue that taking consent is irrelevant, as they would not be expected to do so in actual clinical practise. Although it is true that you are unlikely to take consent for a hernia operation as a house officer, this is probably because of lack of opportunities and eagerness on both the part of yourself and your senior. Needless to say, you are obtaining consent during the majority of your working day, whenever you do a procedure, be it urinary catheterisation or intravenous cannulation or something more technical such as central line insertion. The underlying principles of taking consent are the same, and it is these principles that are being tested.

In most circumstances, gaining a patient's verbal (or in some cases implied) consent is sufficient. In other instances, the patient will need to sign a consent form stating receipt of all the information required for consent and confirmation to go ahead with the proposed procedure. But by no case is this document legally binding, even once signed the patient can still decide not to go ahead with the procedure.

The GMC have recently published guidelines on how to and who can take consent. The person taking consent should be qualified and suitably trained as well as have sufficient knowledge of the procedure, including its risk and benefits.

Note that the person does not have to be competent in the procedure. Although ambiguous in its definition, the suitably trained individual may and is probably referring to you, the foundation programme doctor. Learning to take consent is a valuable skill whether you go into surgical training or not.

You will come across gaining consent in many of the OSCE stations, when asked to perform any form of examination, or you will be asked to gain consent for a specific procedure. So it is important you understand the risks and benefits of commonly performed procedures and other invasive investigations in surgery where sufficient knowledge is required at an undergraduate level, or as stipulated in your syllabus.

As with any clinical encounter, do not forget the general principles as outlined above (*see* Principles of a clinical encounter, p. 13).

For purposes of clarity, we have demonstrated the underlying principles using a common procedure you are likely to encounter in the examination.

Case 1: Obtaining consent

Instructions: This man is about to have an elective inguinal hernia repair. Please consent him for the procedure.

<u>Key features to look out for:</u>
✔ **Gather information**
- Ask the patient if he knows the diagnosis and what/why he is being prepared for the procedure.

✔ **Confirm patient diagnosis and prognosis if left untreated**
- Explain the diagnosis of an inguinal hernia.
- Use diagrams if necessary, as this is often very helpful and will certainly gain you extra points in the examination.

> ### Examiner's Anecdote
>
> *'She was the first candidate that day to draw a diagram explaining the procedure to the patient. Finally, someone who has clearly been to the pre-operative clinic!'*

- Explain the natural history of the condition and the possibility of incarceration and strangulation.

✔ **Outline the treatment options**

- **Option not to treat:** Patient has absolute autonomy and can refuse for any reason, unless incompetent. You must explain the consequences of not accepting treatment.
- **Options for treatment:** You must discuss all the viable treatment options available for the patient. This includes conservative, medical or surgical options and their associated risks and benefits.
- **Treatment of choice:** You should be able to tell the patient the treatment of choice for the condition. If there is a better treatment available elsewhere, the patient should be informed of this, according to GMC guidelines. Ideally the treatment of choice is the one being offered, but this may not always be the case.
- **Treatment being offered:** *See below.*
- **Right to second opinion:** Patients can seek a second opinion from an independent consultant if they wish.

✔ **Discuss the proposed treatment**

- **Name the procedure:** Use the correct medical terms, and then explain them in lay terms.
  - E.g. *'Elective open repair of a left inguinal hernia'.*
- **Doctor who retains overall responsibility:** This is typically the consultant in charge, but also mention that there will be a team involved often with input from complementary specialities, i.e. the anaesthetist, clinical nurse specialists, etc.
- **The indications:** Explain why the patient is being offered this over another more common procedure, i.e. there may be a contraindication to the treatment of choice.
- **Relative benefits:** you must also explain the probability of a successful procedure.
  - E.g. *'To reduce associated symptoms such as discomfort or pain and to prevent the occurrence of complications (risk of incarceration and strangulation)'.*
- **Outline of procedure:** Describe this in layman's terms, using diagrams as appropriate; if the procedure is experimental or part of a research study, then this must be included.
- **Use of any subsidiary treatment:** This depends on the case but in general, patients would like to know if they will require a urinary catheter or an epidural postoperatively, so make sure you inform them of this as appropriate.
- **Discuss preoperative and postoperative care:** Discuss the preoperative planning, such as stopping Warfarin, the need for keeping NBM, and so on. Explain what the patient should expect postoperatively, i.e. whether they will be in HDU or will go straight to the ward, when they can eat, drink and mobilise. Usually the anaesthetist will be able to discuss this in more detail

with the patient. Patients are keen to know when they will be discharged home, so give them an estimated time. Also at this time, take the opportunity to explain any follow-up arrangements and contact details in case of complications, e.g. the GP, district nurse care or clinic appointments.

■ **Risks and side effects:** You must inform your patient of any serious or frequently occurring risks, including any common and serious side effects – preferably with a nationally recognised probability of occurrence – but ideally using the operating surgeon's or surgical centre's own figures. If the procedure will result in significant lifestyle changes you must inform the patient (e.g. not being able to work for a certain period of time after the procedure).

Table 1.6: Inguinal hernia repair complications

Complications	Examples
General surgical	Pain, infection (both wound and mesh, later LRTI, urinary), bleeding, DVT/PE.
Specific complications to hernia repair	Recurrence requiring further surgery, chronic pain or numbness in the groin (as a result of damage to the ilioinguinal nerve).
	Reduced fertility, testicular atrophy or formation of a varicocele (this occurs as a result of damage to the cord structures including the vas, testicular artery and the pampiniform plexus of veins; it is very important you explain this to a male patient who is still thinking of having a family, as it can result in infertility).
	Damage to the bladder or bowel (which may be part of the hernial contents).
	Urinary retention post-operatively requiring a catheter (secondary to the pain).
	Haematoma or seroma formation.

✔ **Consent for supplemental/unforeseen procedures**
  ■ **Acceptable procedures:** Should an unexpected but well-recognised complication arise intraoperatively there may not be enough time to wake the patient and obtain valid consent to deal with the problem. This is particularly important with regards to the use of blood transfusions or bowel resection in the case of an exploratory laparotomy. You must therefore establish what supplemental procedures the patient will consent for should this situation arise.
  ■ **Unacceptable procedures:** Ascertain the procedures the patient will refuse under any circumstances, e.g. blood transfusion, and document this very clearly, stating the reason.
✔ **Check for valid consent**
  ■ **Capacity for consent:** Ascertain whether the patient has understood your explanation and can make a decision. Legally you must demonstrate the following:
    – **Understands information:** Has the patient understood what you have said in a language he understands?

- **Retains information:** Is he able to remember the information long enough to cognitively process and come up with a decision?
- **Makes a decision:** Is he able to weigh up the information, its risk and benefits, and make a decision?
- **Communicates that decision:** Is he able to communicate the decision to you either verbally (in any language), non-verbally (including gestures and sign language) or through written communication (i.e. a signed consent form)?

Competence is a legal definition; the capacity to consent can be determined by any physician. A mentally disabled patient may still have the capacity to consent even if the reasons for refusal seem irrational.

Authors' Top Tip

Remember, autonomy is absolute and every patient is deemed competent unless you have reason to think otherwise or a court of law has told you so.

- **Respond to any questions:** You must ensure you give the patient an opportunity to ask questions. If you do not know the answer, be honest and say you will find out.

Examiner's Anecdote

'Do not make up answers to a patient's question; it is okay if you don't know the answer, we will not hold this against you, so long as you tell the patient you will find out the answer once you've spoken to your senior colleagues. We are testing your communication skills and not necessarily your detailed knowledge of complication occurrence rates. If you make something up, your professional integrity will be questioned and consequently you will be negatively marked.'

✔ **Confirm patient's right to withdraw consent**
- **Patient retains absolute autonomy:** the patient may refuse consent at any point, even in the anaesthetic room. The refusal does not have to be verbal. You must inform patients of this right, should they later say that they were not aware they could refuse at any point, even on the operating table.

Completion

You must ensure you give the patient an opportunity to ask questions, and if you do not know the answer, be honest and say you will find out.

The most common cause for liability in surgical practise is when a patient claims the consent was not valid. A signed document does not necessarily absolve you from any wrongdoing. Even in cases where patients refuse to consent for your proposed treatment, they can still hold you accountable for invalid consent if you did not explain the risks of them not agreeing to your treatment option. For example, if a patient needs a coronary angioplasty after having suffered an MI, and you explain that the procedure has a significant risk of bleeding – and the patient refused treatment on this basis and subsequently died – legally you are still held accountable, as you did not explain the consequences of not going through with the treatment. The patient's representative could then argue that had the patient known of the risk of death associated with refusing consent for treatment, he would have consented for the original intended procedure and so the original consent you obtained was invalid!

Authors' Top Tip

We strongly recommend you follow the detailed GMC guidelines on consent through-out your professional careers and accurately document your consultation in the notes.

Explaining a procedure

Information-giving OSCE stations where the principles of explaining a procedure (or an investigation) are commonly tested in finals. Clearly, you must be aware of the principles of the procedure itself and be able to communicate this accurately to the patient.

Authors' Top Tip

Visit the endoscopy and radiology departments of your teaching hospitals where numerous patient leaflets are available explaining the commonly performed outpatient procedures. The outlines used in these leaflets are very similar to how you will be marked in the actual examination.

Although similar to consent, this station is best approached in a question/answer format in which the most common questions a patient will have are answered as part of your discussion. Below we have provided all the information in layman's terms regarding gastroscopy and the types of questions your patient may ask you.

Remember, as with all patient consultations, always bear in mind the general principles and communication skills that you need to demonstrate throughout the encounter; these will score you a great deal of marks.

Case 2: Explain a procedure

Instructions: This woman is about to undergo a gastroscopy; please explain the procedure to her.

Key features to look out for:
✔ Gather information
- Ascertain whether the patient knows the diagnosis and the procedure she is being prepared for and why.
- Ask how much the patient knows already and how much she would like to know.

✔ **Outline the proposed procedure**
- ■ **What is a gastroscopy?**
  - – 'A gastroscopy is where a thin, flexible, fibre-optic instrument containing a video camera and light source at one end is passed through your mouth, down your gullet, through your stomach and into the first part of your small bowel, called the duodenum.
  - – The instrument looks like a long, thin tube and is about three feet long; it is approximately the diameter of your small finger.
  - – It is passed into your mouth through a teeth guard while you lie down on your left side. Once the instrument is placed into your mouth you are asked to swallow it; this is the part that most patients find uncomfortable.
  - – Once the instrument reaches the stomach, the endoscopist may need to pump some air into the stomach. This may be a little uncomfortable and gives you the sensation that you need to burp.
  - – During the procedure, biopsies may be taken; these will be painless.
  - – A gastroscopy allows the examination of the lining of these structures.
  - – As the instrument makes its journey, the images are displayed in real time to the endoscopist on a TV screen in front of him or her. This will allow a further course of treatment or investigation to be initiated if necessary.
  - – In general, the examination should last up to 15 mins'.
- ■ **What are the associated risks or complications?**
  - – 'All procedures carry risks; although minor complications do occur, they are not common and major complications are rare.
  - – In general, the associated complications are discomfort during the procedure and some slight throat soreness afterwards for a day or so. There is a small risk of infection.
  - – If biopsies are taken, there is a very small risk that the site will continue to bleed, and there is also a small chance of causing a perforation (hole) in the stomach or gullet; both of the latter complications may require an operation'.

✔ **Outline all available options**
- ■ **Are there any alternatives?**
  - – 'Yes, X-rays with barium, but these will not allow for an examination of the lining of the stomach or allow for biopsies to be taken so important things may be missed'.

✔ **Discuss pre-procedure care**
- ■ **What happens before the test?**
  - – 'You will not be allowed to eat or drink for 4–6 hours immediately prior to the procedure, because the stomach needs to be empty.
  - – If you are taking any medications for indigestion you may be asked to stop taking these at least two weeks before the procedure'.
- ■ **What happens on the day of the test?**
  - – 'On the day of the test, or sometimes during your outpatient consultation, you will be asked to sign a consent form for the procedure, stating you understand the risks, complications, benefits and alternatives of the procedure'.

✔ Discuss peri-procedure care
  ■ **Is it painful?**
    – *'The procedure is painless, although you may find it is slightly uncomfortable'.*
  ■ **Will I be awake during the procedure?**
    – *'Light sedation may be offered to you; if so, you will still be awake during the procedure.*
    – *Some people elect to undergo the procedure without any sedation, in which case the back of your throat is sprayed with some local anaesthetic'.*
✔ Discuss post-procedure care
  ■ **Will I be kept in hospital for the test?**
    – *'It is done as a day case, and you can normally go home following the procedure.*
    – *If you have had sedation, then you will need another responsible adult with you, as you are not allowed to drive or operate heavy machinery for at least 24 hours.*
    – *If you have had the local anaesthetic to the back of the throat, then you should not have anything to eat or drink for one hour after the procedure'.*
✔ Inform the patient of follow-up arrangements
  ■ **When will I be told the results?**
    – *'The doctor or nurse may talk to you after the procedure to tell you the findings, although if you have had some light sedation you may still be drowsy after the procedure and may not remember the procedure at all.*
    – *If biopsies have been taken, then it takes a few days to get the results'.*

Completion

You must ensure that you give the patient an opportunity to ask questions. If you do not know the answer, be honest and say that you will speak to a senior who knows and will get back to the patient.

The content of the above case is just an example and can be adjusted to a clinical scenario. We suggest you read your syllabus regarding other possible investigations you are required to know and prepare for them appropriately.

(
_____

Taking a surgical history

It is often said that the medical student history is thorough, detailed and comprehensive. However, in actual clinical practice you may find that time is very limited, preventing you from taking such a detailed and thorough history. The objective should be to identify the salient points needed to reach an accurate diagnosis. The best way to gauge how much information is required during the history-taking process is to present as often as the opportunity arises, preferably to a surgical consultant during a post-take ward round. Unfortunately, with the advent of the EWTD, you may find yourself in a situation where you are not present for the post-take ward round after having finished an evening or night on call. This makes it even more important that you take and document a concise and clear history, as your history will most likely be read and interpreted by one of your colleagues. Your train of thought must be obvious to your colleague.

We advise being systematic but concise to illicit the relevant negative and positive points during the history-taking process. Your aim should be to take a focused history, in a busy environment such as the A&E department, within a set period of time. The time allowed for a history-taking station during the OSCE can range from 5 to 20 minutes, depending on your particular medical school. For those of you who think taking a history in five minutes is not possible, one of the author's third-year OSCEs involved doing just that. Although challenging, it is certainly possible, as long as you ask focused and clinically relevant questions.

We therefore describe focused clinical histories, most commonly seen in an acute surgical setting. Being focused does not equate to being rude or sharp with your patient. This attitude will not stand in your favour, therefore be tactful when dealing with the patient who is veering off topic and direct the conversation, but do not dictate it.

Authors' Top Tip

Do not forget that many marks are to be gained by demonstrating your communication skills as well as the rapport you build with your patient during the short time you have.

Surgical history

General principles
✔ Introduce yourself and confirm that you are talking to the right patient
✔ Explain purpose of meeting; gain consent

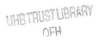

✔ **Communication skills pertinent to history-taking**
  - **Physical setting:** You should be seated at the same level as the patient, with no physical barriers such as a large table between you and the patient.
  - **Question formats:** Start the conversation with an open-ended question, then move on to closed questions, if needed. Avoid asking single answer, yes or no, questions.
  - **Non-verbal communication:** Use appropriate gestures to maintain a friendly and attentive persona. Respond to nonverbal cues as appropriate.
  - **Verbal communication:** React to the patient's concerns and expectations; try to be empathic where appropriate. Periodically make use of summaries and signposting, as this helps clarify any queries the patient may have and the opportunity to add new information. This also provides you with a chance to think of any further questions you may want to ask to complete your history. Make good use of natural pauses in the conversation for this purpose.

The history

✔ **Presenting complaint**
✔ **History of presenting complaint** (*see below for specific cases*)
✔ **Past medical/surgical history/family history**
  - Check for any pre-existing medical conditions.
  - Is there a history of previous hospitalisations or operations?
✔ **Drug history and allergies**
  - In the OSCE you may not have time to take a detailed list of all medications and dosages, but ensure you check for any allergic reactions.
✔ **Systems review**
  - There are often associated symptoms that occur commonly with the presenting complaint.
  - This also serves to form the basis of useful negative or positive symptoms that may help to differentiate between the various differential diagnoses.
  - For example, in the case of abdominal pain, it is prudent to ask if the patient has jaundice, as this will help focus your attention to the liver and biliary tree.
✔ **Risk factors assessment**
  - This can be a very useful signpost in the exam. For example, whilst taking a history of a breast lump, you can inform the patient that you would now like to assess for risk factors of breast cancer. In doing so, you are also informing the examiner of what you are doing next and your intention.
  - This can be adapted to almost any presenting complaint and these are a list of important features that help you to assess the severity of a patient's diagnosis.
✔ **Social history**
  - **Occupation**
  - **Smoking and alcohol intake:** This is usually related to risk factor assessment.
  - **Home situation:** The ability to perform the normal activities of daily living. Enquire whether the patient lives in a ground or top floor apartment, as this is important to assess when deciding whether a patient can cope in his or her own home with the current health issues.

Case 1: Testicular pain

Instructions: This man presents with a history of testicular pain. Please take a focused clinical history.

Key features to look for:
✔ **Note the patient's age**
  ■ The patient's age group can help differentiate the cause in order of likelihood:

Table 2.1: Testicular pain age groups

Age group	Aetiology
Prepubertal	Mumps orchitis, idiopathic scrotal oedema, testicular torsion
Adolescent (10–21 years)	Testicular torsion (most likely), epididymo-orchitis, torsion of the Hydatid of Morgagni (7–14 years)
Adult (>21 years)	Epididymo-orchitis (most likely), testicular torsion
All age groups	Trauma

✔ **Testicular pain**
  ■ **Site:** Is the pain unilateral or bilateral? Bilateral testicular pain is seen in mumps orchitis, whereas unilateral is typically seen in testicular torsion and epididymo-orchitis.
  ■ **Onset:** Acute onset within hours can be either testicular torsion or epididymo-orchitis, although the latter tends to have a more gradual mode of onset that can last several days.
  ■ **Character:** A sharp, unrelenting pain is more likely to be testicular torsion, whereas a dull ache that feels heavy may be epididymo-orchitis.
  ■ **Radiation:** Pain in testicular origin can be referred to the thigh, groin or the abdomen as the testicles share T10 dermatome; pain extending to the penile shaft or perineum can occur in idiopathic scrotal oedema.
  ■ **Alleviating factors:** Pain that is relieved on standing up or wearing scrotal support that elevates the testicles suggests epididymo-orchitis.
  ■ **Timing:** The pain is usually constant in both testicular torsion and epididymo-orchitis; colicky pain should prompt you to consider alternative diagnoses such as ureteric colic, which can lead to referred testicular pain.
  ■ **Exacerbating factors:** The pain can occur acutely after a history of trauma or trivial exertion, e.g. exercise or sexual intercourse.
  ■ **Scale:** Exquisite tenderness suggests torsion, whereas epididymo-orchitis tends to be less painful; mumps orchitis and scrotal oedema typically display a low-grade discomfort.
✔ **Associated symptoms**
  ■ **Urinary symptoms:** Dysuria, urinary frequency and urethral discharge are commonly seen in epididymo-orchitis; characteristically, testicular torsion has no urinary symptoms.

- **Sexual history:** This is an important aspect of the history, particularly in an adolescent, as chlamydia or gonorrhoea can cause epididymo-orchitis. The general points to illicit include any recent history of sexual intercourse, whether he has had a regular partner or a new partner, whether he uses condoms and lastly if he has noticed urethral discharge. (Please note that this is not an exhaustive list for taking a sexual history.)
- **Swelling:** Swelling and erythema of the scrotal skin suggest scrotal oedema or mumps orchitis. Swelling that occurs soon after trauma suggests a haematoma. It is important to note that swelling can occur in torsion as well.
- **Fever/vomiting:** Fever can occur with epididymo-orchitis, torsion or mumps orchitis. Although not specific to torsion, patients may vomit because of the unrelenting pain.

✔ **Medical history**
- **Previous history:** Patients who have testicular torsion usually have had previous episodes of testicular pain – the so-called intermittent torsion, where the testis twists on its mesentery but spontaneously untwists.
- **History of mumps:** Patients who have recently suffered from parotitis can also develop a viral orchitis that can cause bilateral testicular pain for up to a week after initial infection.

Completion

You are almost certainly not going to get a case of testicular torsion in the examination; what the examiners are looking for is that you have considered testicular torsion as your main differential, because it is a surgical emergency. For more information on scrotal examination: (*see* Chapter 7, Testicular lumps).

Viva questions

Q1   What investigations would you request?
- Usually none are required if torsion is suspected on clinical grounds.
- The patient will need to be taken to a theatre within six hours of symptom onset to avoid irreversible ischaemia and testicular infarction.
- In equivocal cases where imaging will not delay the patient from going to a theatre, a Doppler USS Testes can be done to assess blood flow into the testicle.
- Otherwise, if time permits, routine preoperative FBC and U&E can be done.
- The following may be helpful:
  - **Urinalysis:** leucocytes to check for pyuria.
  - **Urine sample:** for MC&S; looking specifically for *E. coli*.
  - **Urethral swab:** screen for sexually transmitted infections.

Epididymo-orchitis can occur in any age group, although it is uncommon in adolescents. If patients present with signs and symptoms suggestive of this diagnosis, the causative organism is usually a sexually transmitted infection, most commonly gonorrhoea and chlamydia. In the very young and older adult age groups the causative organism is *E. coli*.

Q2   How would you differentiate testicular torsion from epididymo-orchitis?

(Difficult Question)

Table 2.2: Torsion versus epididymo-orchitis

Variable	Epididymo-orchitis	Testicular torsion
Onset	Gradual onset (hours to days).	Acute onset (hours).
Age	Usually in an older age group or young sexually active males.	Adolescent boys (10–16 years).
Urinary symptoms	Dysuria and frequency; there may be urethral discharge in STI.	None.
History	Uncommon.	Episodes of previous testicular pain are common (intermittent torsion).
Examination findings	Fever, tender epididymis and/or testes, positive Prehn's sign *(see below)*.	Exquisitely tender/swollen testicle, high-riding testicle in scrotum, Bell Clapper Deformity (testicle is lying horizontally), absent cremasteric reflex.
Urinalysis	Pyuria, STI on urethral swabs.	Normal.
Doppler USS Testes	Increased blood flow in epididymis.	Reduced or absent blood flow.

Prehn's sign is said to be positive when elevation of the testes with the patient in a supine position relieves the testicular pain. This is not seen in testicular torsion. The pain in torsion is mainly testicular in site, although it may radiate to the groin or abdomen. The use of Doppler USS in equivocal cases can aid in diagnosis, where you will see poor flow through the testicular artery, indicating torsion; increased blood flow through the epididymis suggests epididymo-orchitis. Here, it must be mentioned that this is operator-dependent, but in experienced hands USS can be up to 80% sensitive and 85% specific. Imaging should not delay any definite operative management.

Q3   Aside from testicular torsion and epididymo-orchitis, what other conditions can cause acute testicular pain?

(Difficult Question)

Table 2.3: Differential diagnosis of testicular pain

Differential	Description
Torsion of the Hydatid of Morgagni	This tends to occur in males between 7 and 14 years of age and can be gradual in onset. The pain is not as severe as that of testicular torsion, and the patient has urinary symptoms with less scrotal swelling. Classically you see the 'blue dot' sign at the upper pole of the testis, which is felt as a palpable tender nodule on clinical examination. It is very difficult to distinguish between testicular torsion, and so most patients undergo operative management where the diagnosis of a torted Hydatid of Morgagni is made.

(Continued)

Table 2.3: Differential diagnosis of testicular pain (*Continued*)

Differential	Description
Mumps orchitis	Prepubertal males who have developed mumps parotitis can develop bilateral orchitis, leading to swelling and pain in both testicles up to a week after the initial viral infection. The patient usually has a clear history of mumps infection as well as the associated symptoms of fever, malaise and myalgia. It is managed conservatively with simple analgesia, as most cases resolve spontaneously.
Idiopathic scrotal oedema	This occurs in very young children and is thought to be allergic in origin. It involves only the scrotal skin, which appears swollen and erythematous bilaterally, but can extend into the penile shaft and perineum. It is important to note that the testicles and epididymis are usually not affected. This is managed conservatively with supportive measures.
Trauma	Trauma is usually evident from the history. An USS testes is useful to differentiate between a haematoma, which is managed conservatively, and testicular rupture, which needs operative treatment.
Tumour	Although an unusual presentation, 10% of testicular malignancies can present acutely with pain. This will often be an incidental finding on USS testes, and the patient requires an urgent referral to the urologist for an orchidectomy.

Case 2: Breast lump

Instructions: A woman presents with a swelling in her breast. Please take a focused clinical history.

Key features to look for:
- **Swellings:** Does it involve the whole breast, or is there a localised lump? Swelling of the whole breast suggests mastitis, lactation or pregnancy. Is the swelling related to the menstrual cycle, i.e. cyclical?
- **Palpable lump:** Can the patient feel the lump?
  - **Site:** Where is the lump in the breast? Upper outer quadrant lumps are more likely to be malignant.
  - **Tenderness:** Is the lump tender, and is the tenderness associated with the woman's menstrual cycle? A breast abscess is typically painful but non-cyclical. Cyclical pain tends to be benign. Cysts can be painful. Malignant lumps are often painless.
  - **Duration:** When was it first noticed, and how long has the lump been there?
  - **Number of lumps:** Ask if the patient has noticed more than one lump, and where in the breast they are located. Are there lumps elsewhere? Lumps in the axilla are probably enlarged regional lymph nodes. Multiple lumps could be multiple cysts or fibroadenomas.
  - **Changes in size:** Has the lump increased or decreased in size over time?

- **Relationship to menstrual cycle:** Does the lump change with cyclicity; if so, how? Does the breast get more lumpy and tender as the period approaches? If pre-menopausal, when was the last menstrual cycle?
- **Special characteristics:**
  - ❑ **Associations:** Did the lump occur post-trauma? If so, fat necrosis is likely.
  - ❑ **Mobile:** Is the lump fairly mobile, as seen in fibroadenomas?
  - ❑ **Skin changes:** Ask about surrounding eczema and whether this is unilateral or bilateral; this could be a sign of Paget's disease of the breast.
  - ❑ **Nipple changes:** Is there any retraction of the nipple as seen in cancer?. Has she noticed any discharge, and if so what colour is it? (*See below*)
- **Discharge:** Has the patient experienced any discharge from the lump; if so, is this bilateral or unilateral; what colour is it? Is there any relation to the menstrual period (cyclical)?

Table 2.4: Breast discharge

Colour	Possible diagnosis
Bloody	Ductal papilloma, intraductal carcinoma, Paget's disease
Clear	Intraductal papilloma
Yellow/green	Duct ectasia
Purulent	Abscess
Milky	Galactorrhoea secondary to hyperprolactinaemia

- **Alarm symptoms:** These are related to metastatic spread of breast cancer. Therefore, it is important to ask about bone pain, particularly back pain, which may be due to pathological fractures or metastatic deposits on the spine; also ask whether she has noticed any weight loss or breathlessness (this is usually secondary to the development of a pleural effusion from pulmonary metastases).
- **Risk factor assessment:** Enquire about the risk factors that increase the risk of developing breast cancer.

Table 2.5: Breast cancer risk factors

Risk factor	Description
Family history	**First-degree relative:** Family history of breast cancer in a first-degree relative; the risk is increased if the relative(s) developed breast cancer under the age of 50 years. **Close relatives:** Increased risk if two close relatives were diagnosed with breast cancer under 50 years of age.

(*Continued*)

Table 2.5: Breast cancer risk factors (*Continued*)

Risk factor	Description
	Male breast cancer: Increased risk if there is a family history of male breast cancer; inheritance is linked to the BRCA 1 (also associated with increased risk of ovarian carcinoma) and BRCA 2 (also linked with increased risk of prostate, bladder and pancreas) genes, which are autosomal dominant with variable penetration, although they are responsible for <5% of breast cancers.
Age	**Increasing age:** Increasing risk with increasing age; however, when diagnosed in young women, the cancers are often more aggressive with a poorer prognosis.
Exposure to oestrogens	**Age of menarche/menopause:** Early menarche (<11 yrs); late menopause (>51 yrs), i.e. greater length of exposure to oestrogen. **Number of pregnancies:** Nulliparous. **Age at first pregnancy:** First birth after the age of 30 years. **Use of oral contraceptive pill (OCP):** OCP use for a period greater than four years before first pregnancy. **Use of HRT:** HRT usage risk is linked to the duration of treatment. Risk rises significantly after >10 years usage of HRT, and risk is substantially higher when using combination oestrogen-progesterone HRT as opposed to oestrogen HRT on its own.
Breastfeeding	**History of breastfeeding:** A history of breastfeeding does not increase risk; it is protective.
Breast cancer	**History of breast cancer:** Does the patient have a prior history of breast cancer in the same or opposite breast?
Exposure to carcinogens	**Radiation exposure:** History of chest radiation in the previous 20 years; this would normally have been received as lymphoma treament.

Completion

The majority of breast lumps are benign; however, all women should undergo triple assessment to rule out malignancy. In your differential diagnosis, always remember that lumps anywhere on the body, including the breast, could be a sebaceous cyst or lipoma. For more information on breast examination: (*see* Chapter 5, Breast).

Viva questions

Q1   What is the differential diagnosis of a breast lump?

Table 2.6: Causes of a breast lump

Differential	Description
Cyst	A benign, fluid-filled collection that is smooth, soft and may be fluctuant. If you are palpating a tense breast cyst, it may not be fluctuant. A cyst usually disappears after aspiration, but if there is a residual lump this will need further investigation. Cysts may be multiple and are common in perimenopausal women. They are the commonest cause of breast lumps in those between 30 and 50 years of age.
Fibroadenoma	Hard, firm and mobile lump, known as 'breast mice'. These occur as a result of excess growth of glandular and connective tissue and may disappear on their own. It is the commonest cause of a breast lump in those <35 years. Note that there is no risk of progression to malignancy.
Breast cancer	These are characteristically hard lumps with an irregular surface.
Intraductal papilloma	A benign lump, usually occurring near the nipples in the sub-areolar ducts; may also cause nipple discharge.
Breast pseudo lumps	These benign lumps are caused by: i. Scar tissue; hardened silicone. ii. Necrotic fat commonly secondary to trauma, giving a hard irregular mass that is difficult to distinguish between carcinoma, although this often decreases in size over time.
Fibrocystic disease – 'fibroadenosis'	A benign condition that physiologically changes in size with the menstrual cycle, being most lumpy premenstrually. This causes lumpiness and tenderness, commonly in the upper outer quadrant.
Lipoma	This may change the shape of the breast; it is benign.
Abscess	Presents as tenderness, erythema and localised swelling. Common in patients who are breastfeeding, secondary to *staphylococcus aureus* infection. It is also seen in non-lactating women, where it is termed 'periductal mastitis'. The abscess is treated by aspiration under USS guidance.
Hamartoma	Could be detected incidentally on mammography; classically described as looking like 'a breast within a breast' due to the composition of breast lobules, stroma and fat enclosed by a capsule.
Phyllodes tumour	Group of neoplasms ranging from benign to malignant with similar characteristics to fibro adenomas.

Q2 How is Li-Fraumeni syndrome linked to breast cancer?

(Honours Question)

- Through the mutation of the p53 gene, inherited in an AD fashion. Individuals are more susceptible to the development of particular cancers, and this includes breast cancer, amongst others.
- This disorder is seen in 1% of early-age breast cancer cases and 25% of cases in those with bilateral breast cancer.

Case 3: Intermittent claudication

Instructions: This man presents with calf pain on walking. Please take a focused clinical history.

Key features to look for:
- **Assess the pain regarding:**
  - **Site:** The extent of the leg pain can help in determining the degree of arterial disease. Calf pain is typically femoral in origin, whereas pain extending into the buttocks suggests arterial occlusive disease is present more proximally, involving the aorto-iliac vessels. Comparatively, pain in a dermatomal distribution is likely to be spinal stenosis.
  - **Onset:** If the pain occurs gradually on walking, then this is more likely to be arterial disease, as opposed to the sudden onset of pain experienced in spinal stenosis, which may or may not be related to walking.
  - **Character:** Intermittent claudication is classically described as an ache or cramp-like pain. Paraesthesiae and numbness are more prominent features of spinal stenosis.
  - **Radiation:** If pain radiates to the back, think of spinal claudication.
  - **Alleviating factors:** Does he have to stop walking and rest to make the pain go away? This is known as the claudication distance. If the patient has to sit down to alleviate the pain, this suggests spinal stenosis, or if the patient can simply stand in one place and wait until the pain is gone, then it is more likely to be arterial disease.
  - **Timing:** The pain of intermittent claudication tends to occur when walking up to a particular distance (the claudication distance) and is relieved gradually when the patient stops walking as muscle ischaemia is relieved; compared to spinal claudication, where the pain is rapid in onset and is not relieved by rest unless the patient coincidentally sits down.
  - **Exacerbating factors:** Is the pain worse when walking (particularly uphill in intermittent claudication)?
  - **Scale:** As with all symptoms of pain, it is useful to gauge the degree of pain on a scale of 1–10. Some patients with intermittent claudication can walk through the pain and develop a collateral blood supply.
- **Assess disease severity:**
  - **Claudication distance:** This is the distance the patient can walk until he must stop walking because of the pain. This pain is due to muscle ischaemia, secondary to arterial disease. The distance is remarkably consistent, and even after resting the patient will often walk the same distance again until he has to rest for the second time. Take note of the actual distance for two reasons: a progressively reducing distance could be a sign of worsening disease, and the actual distance itself will

help assess the patient's social care needs – particularly if the patient cannot walk to the shops due to pain.

- **Rest pain:** If the patient experiences the same pain when he is at rest, this is a sign of critical ischaemia (stage III fontaine).
- **Night pain:** This is essentially rest pain, but at night. A classical description is that patients must swing their legs out of bed to get relief. This is because gravity will increase the blood supply to the dependent limb, alleviating the ischaemia. For this reason, ask if the patient sleeps in a chair, as this keeps the legs dependent.
- **Ulcers:** Ask the patient if he has noticed any ulcers or skin changes to his legs; these may suggest a diagnosis of peripheral vascular disease. Ask about the location of these ulcers and whether they are painful, which will help you to work out whether they are arterial or venous in origin. Ulceration is a sign of critical ischaemia (*see* Chapter 9, Examination of ulcers).

■ **Risk factor assessment:** There are several risk factors for developing atherosclerotic disease; specifically ask about the following:
- Diabetes, smoking, obesity, age (>50 years).
- Hypercholesterolaemia, hypertension.

■ **Associated symptoms:**
- **Sexual history:** In a male patient, it is important to ask about impotence, as this could be a sign of Leriche's syndrome, where aorto-iliac arterial disease leads to buttock claudication, atrophy and erectile dysfunction.
- **Medical history:** If the patient is a known arteriopath (particularly if they have had previous CVAs/TIAs/MI/angina/AF), then a diagnosis of arterial disease is more likely.

Completion

There are a number of differential diagnoses, but for purposes of finals arterial disease is the most likely cause, and the examiner would like to see you emphasise this in your answer. An important differential to exclude is spinal stenosis, which can cause spinal claudication, mimicking the symptoms of intermittent claudication.

Table 2.7: Differential diagnosis of calf pain

Classification	Cause
Arterial disease	Arterial occlusive disease, popliteal entrapment syndrome
Neurological	Spinal stenosis, peripheral neuropathy, lumbar radiculopathy
Orthopaedic	Plantar fasciitis, compartment syndrome
Chronic venous	Post-phlebitic limb, chronic venous insufficiency
Medical	Rheumatoid arthritis, osteoarthritis, vasculitis

For more information on peripheral arterial disease *see* Chapter 9.

Viva questions

Q1 Why is rest pain classically felt at night?

(Difficult Question)

- In the recumbent position, the beneficial effects of gravity are lost in the lower limb.
- Therefore perfusion, in addition to cardiac output, BP and HR, are all reduced when we sleep, as there is lower metabolic demand.
- Decreased perfusion leads to muscle ischaemia in a patient with severe arterial disease, and consequently pain at night.

Q2 What is the Fontaine Classification System?

(Honours Question)

In 1954, Dr Rene Fontaine introduced the four stages used in the classification of peripheral arterial disease:

Table 2.8: Fontaine classification

Stage	Description
1	**Claudication:** Pain in the calf brought on by walking; resulting from muscle ischaemia.
2	**Intermittent claudication**: Pain brought on by walking short distances due to arterial insufficiency and relieved by rest.
3	**Rest pain/critical ischaemia:** Burning pain in the forefoot that is brought on by elevation and relieved by dependency. Rest pain is ischaemia of muscles as well as soft tissues; usually experienced by the patient at night and relieved by hanging the foot over the side of the bed.
4	**Tissue loss (gangrene/ulceration)**: The consequences of severe occlusive arterial disease.

Authors' Top Tip

The history you take should help illicit symptoms that will classify the degree of peripheral arterial disease. The top students can then grade this and mention the likely grading when they present their history to the examiner.

Q3 How would you differentiate between intermittent claudication due to peripheral vascular disease and spinal claudication due to spinal stenosis?

Table 2.9: Vascular versus spinal stenosis

Variable	Vascular	Spinal
Onset	Pain is gradual on movement and relieved by rest	Rapid onset of pain, worse on movement, not relieved by rest
History of PAD	Yes	No
Pain distribution	Calf, buttocks	Dermatomal
Aetiology	Chronic vascular insufficiency	Nerve compression

Q4   How would you differentiate between a thrombotic cause and an embolic cause of acute limb ischaemia?

Table 2.10: Embolic versus thrombotic

Variable	Embolic cause	Thrombotic cause
Onset	Minutes	Hours
Affected site	Can be multiple areas	Usually a specific limb
History of PAD	Can be none	Usually signs of chronic vascular insufficiency on the affected side
Claudication	No previous history	Usually has claudication or rest pain
History	Recent MI, AF	Known arteriopath

Q5   What is an emergency embolectomy, and what was Thomas Fogarty famous for?

(Difficult Question)

- During an embolectomy, the femoral artery on the side of the symptomatic leg is exposed and a thin, flexible catheter (Fogarty catheter) with a deflated balloon at the end of it is guided as far down the vessel as possible.
- The balloon is then inflated and is slowly withdrawn, pulling the embolus with it. The artery is then closed.
- Thomas Fogarty was a medical student who designed this ingenious piece of equipment.

Q6   How does someone with a DVT (which is present in the venous system) get a PE (located in the arterial system)?
- This is the so-called 'paradoxical embolus'.
- The DVT travels through a cardiac septal defect into the arterial circulation, causing a pulmonary embolus.

Case 4: Rectal bleeding

Instructions: This man presents with rectal bleeding. Please take a focused clinical history.

Key features to look for:
- **Assess rectal blood:** The features associated with bleeding can aid in the diagnosis.
  - **Pain:** The presence of pain or anal irritation is a useful distinguishing feature.
    - Painful bleeding typically occurs in anal canal pathology, such as anal fissures. The exception is haemorrhoids, which are almost always painless. More proximal colonic pathology causing bleeding is usually painless.

- ❑ Pain that is relieved on defecation suggests IBD or irritable bowel syndrome.
- – **Colour of blood:**
  - ❑ **Bright red:** Suggests anal canal bleeding, such as haemorrhoids or polyps.
  - ❑ **Dark red:** May be from more proximal colonic pathology; including an upper GI bleed.
  - ❑ **Black:** Black, tarry stools are likely to be malaena, which occurs in an upper GI bleed due to the breakdown of blood by the acidic contents of the stomach.
- – **Blood pattern:**
  - ❑ **Toilet paper:** If blood is found on the toilet paper after wiping, this is likely to be due to bleeding from the anal canal, e.g. haemorrhoids or anal fissures.
  - ❑ **Faeces:** If the blood is mixed with the stools, then the source of blood is likely to be more proximal, i.e. from the colon, which can be due to IBD.
- – **Amount:** Lower GI bleeding is divided arbitrarily into massive, moderate and occult based on the amount of blood, the patient's hemodynamic status and his or her Hb.
  - ❑ **Massive bleeds:** The patient is usually haemodynamically unstable; these bleeds are torrential and are commonly due to diverticular disease or angiodysplasia. Massive bleeding due to IBD is rare.
  - ❑ **Moderate:** Found in haemodynamically stable patients; these bleeds can be due to benign anorectal conditions or IBD.
  - ❑ **Occult:** These are typically seen in patients with colorectal carcinoma.
- – **Mucous:** Mucous mixed with blood is typically seen in IBD but can also be seen in lesions affecting the colon, such as infective diarrhoea.
- – **Malaena:** Black, tarry stools that occur due to the breakdown of blood in the stomach by its acidic contents. Malaena has a distinctive smell that once encountered will not be forgotten. This is suggestive of an acute upper GI bleed.
- ■ **Change in bowel habit:**
  - – **Increased frequency:** This can be diarrhoea, constipation or alternating episodes of each. If there is increased frequency, it is important to note how many times a day a patient is passing stools, as multiple episodes suggests IBD and >10 times per day is an indication of disease severity.
  - – **Alternating episodes:** Alternating bouts of diarrhoea/constipation suggest IBD.
  - – **Insidious onset:** A more insidious change in bowel habit, particularly in an elderly patient, should prompt you to consider the strong possibility of a colorectal carcinoma, especially when coupled with alarm symptoms such as weight loss or anaemia.

- ■ Colorectal carcinoma risk factor assessment:
  - – Known history of IBD.
  - – Family history of IBD or colorectal cancer.
- ■ **Alarm symptoms:** Anaemia (manifested as tiredness or malaise), weight loss and tenesmus are all suggestive of colorectal carcinoma, but can also be seen in IBD.
- ■ **Associated features:**
  - – **Abdominal pain:** This is particularly important in elderly patients, as this can be a sign of ischaemic colitis; in a younger patient IBD is more likely.
  - – **Foreign travel:** Patients who have recently returned from abroad and have bloody diarrhoea are likely to have infective colitis.
  - – **Change in diet:** This also includes asking about any recent unusual or new food intake, which could indicate food poisoning. Ask if anyone else in the same household has similar symptoms, as again this suggests an infective cause. With infective cases there is usually associated crampy abdominal pain.
  - – **Trauma:** This is an unusual cause of bleeding but can occur if a patient has a history of rectal prolapse that bleeds from repeated trauma.
- ■ **Past medical history:**
  - – **Atrial fibrillation:** An elderly gentleman with AF presenting with abdominal pain or rectal bleeding should immediately prompt you to consider a diagnosis of mesenteric infarction.
  - – **Haematemesis:** A patient who has had a recent history of haematemesis and/or epigastric pain may have had an upper GI bleed, leading to altered digested blood presenting as rectal bleeding.
  - – **Bleeding coagulopathy:** A rare but possible cause of bleeding anywhere in the GI tract.

Authors' Top Tip

Always consider the possibility of a massive upper GI bleed in all patients presenting with a lower GI bleed, as an upper GI bleed has greater morbidity.

- ■ **Drug history:** Patients who are on anticoagulant drugs such as Warfarin or aspirin, especially the elderly, are at increased risk of bleeding, which can be massive. These drugs should be stopped during an acute bleed.

Completion

A similar history can be taken from a patient complaining of a change in bowel habit or a patient referred with concerns that they may have bowel cancer. The important thing to remember is that the key features noted above are the same in either presentation. The important diagnosis not to miss is colorectal carcinoma, and so most patients undergo endoscopic investigation in the form of a flexible sigmoidoscopy or a colonoscopy, which is the gold standard test.

Viva questions

Q1 What signs and symptoms do left- and right-sided colorectal tumours produce?
- **Right-sided:** Iron deficiency anaemia, abdominal mass or pain, diarrhoea.
- **Left-sided:** Change in bowel habit, rectal bleeding, tenesmus; the cancer itself can present with bowel obstruction or perforation.

Most cancers occur in the rectum and sigmoid colon.

Q2 What investigations would you perform in this patient?
- Colonoscopy and Hb.

(Average Response)

In general, the investigations you perform should be tailored to your examination findings (via abdominal examination and DRE) but you may also include the following:
- **Screening test:** In patients whom you suspect that they are having occult bleeding, FOB may be a useful screen.
- **Stool microscopy and cultures:** If suspicious of infective diarrhoea.
- **Blood tests:** FBC for anaemia; haematinics for iron, B12 and folate levels. CRP/ESR if considering IBD. U&Es if considering acute upper GI bleed as a cause, with raised urea a sign of recent bleeding; electrolytes may also be deranged in diarrhoea. LFTs and calcium if considering metastastic spread of colorectal carcinoma to liver and bone respectively. Look for clotting in case the patient is on anticoagulants or has a coagulopathy. Remember to G&S the patient in case he or she needs a blood transfusion.
- **Imaging:** This is usually done to find a cause for the bleeding rather than the source of bleeding. A barium enema can be done to look for signs of IBD, or to look for the characteristic apple core lesion in colorectal carcinoma (*see* Chapter 12, Case 6).
- **Endoscopy and biopsy:** This can help identify the source of bleeding and can be therapeutic. Flexible sigmoidoscopy looks at the whole left colon and rectum, while colonoscopy is reserved for more proximal lesions.

(Good Response)

- **Specialist tests:** If the patient is still bleeding and a source has not been identified, the following may be useful:
  - **Labelled red cell scan:** This test is used in cases where the cause and site of bleeding is undetermined or as a prerequisite to angiography. This is a radionuclide scan that uses red cells labelled with Technetium 99m. These red blood cells then circulate in the blood for 48 hrs and via the use of a gamma camera, which can detect their accumulation and can help identify the site of bleeding. This is useful for conditions such as angiodysplasia, where the bleed rate may be slow but ongoing.
  - **Mesenteric angiogram:** Where extravasation of contrast material can identify the source of bleeding.

(Honours Response)

Q3   What are the causes of rectal bleeding?

Table 2.11: Aetiology of rectal bleeding

Origin	Aetiology
Medical	**Drugs:** Anticoagulants **Haematological:** Blood dyscrasias
Upper GI tract	**Altered digested blood:** Any cause of upper GI bleeding, e.g. bleeding duodenal ulcer
Small bowel	Meckels diverticulum, mesenteric infarction
Colon and rectum	Colorectal carcinoma, diverticular disease, IBD, angiodysplasia, radiation colitis, ischaemic colitis, rectal prolapse, infective colitis
Anal canal	Haemorrhoids, anal fissures, anal carcinoma, trauma

Diverticular disease is an important cause of massive lower GI bleeding. It is an acquired condition of the large bowel, commonly found in the sigmoid colon. It leads to numerous small outpouchings, which occur at areas of weakness in the bowel wall at the point of entry to blood vessels. It is a common condition affecting the Western world, where a low-fibre diet leads to increased intraluminal pressures. Most patients are asymptomatic, but some can present with rectal bleeding, diverticulitis (also known as left-sided appendicitis), bowel obstruction and eventually perforation. For finals purposes, it is important that you do not confuse the nomenclature:

Diverticulae **are outpouchings of the wall of any hollow luminal viscus.**
Diverticulosis **is the presence of diverticulae in the colon.**
Diverticular disease **is the presence of symptomatic diverticulae in the colon.**
Diverticulitis **is the presence of acute inflammation of the diverticulae in the colon.**

(Surgical Definition)

Authors' Top Tip

The diverticulae in diverticular disease are not true diverticulae, as they do not involve all the layers of the bowel wall. An example of a true diverticulum is a Meckel's diverticulum.

A Meckel's diverticulum is a genetic anomaly of the small bowel found in 2% of the population. It is the embryological remnant of the vitelline duct lying on the antimesenteric border of the ileum, two feet (60 cm) from the caecum. It averages two inches (5 cm) in length.

Angiodysplasia is a vascular malformation of unknown cause that occurs sporadically but can be associated with hereditary haemorrhagic telangiectasia. The dilated blood vessels tend to affect the right side of the colon, leading to submucosal vascular swellings that can cause major haemorrhage; therefore, it can be difficult to differentiate this from a diverticular bleed, as diverticular disease is common and the two conditions can therefore coexist. Colonoscopy may find it difficult to identify these lesions, and so in massive bleeds a selective mesenteric angiogram may be helpful, since it characteristically demonstrates a blush lesion in angiodysplasia.

Q4 Can you relate diverticular disease to gallstones?

(Honours Question)

- There is a well-known association called Saint's Triad, where diverticular disease tends to occur with cholelithiasis and a hiatus hernia.

Q5 What is Duke's Classification System?

(Difficult Question)

- It is used to stage colorectal carcinoma

Table 2.12: Duke's Classification

Stage	Description
A	Carcinoma in situ; does not extend into mucosa or submucosa
B1	Tumour extends into muscularis
B2	Tumour extends through serosa
C	Tumour extends to regional lymph nodes
D	Presence of distant metastases

Note that this is a simplified version, suitable for undergraduate purposes; the actual Duke's Staging is far more comprehensive.

Q6 What are the different segments of large bowel?

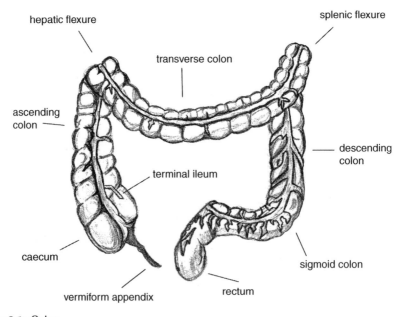

Figure 2.1: Colon

Q7 What are the different bowel resections available for colorectal carcinoma?

(Difficult Question)

Table 2.13: Bowel resections

Operation	Description
Right hemicolectomy	Tumour anywhere from the caecum to the hepatic flexure
Extended right hemicolectomy	Tumour in the transverse colon
Left hemicolectomy	Tumour anywhere distal to the splenic flexure into the descending colon
Anterior resection	**High resection:** Tumour in the sigmoid colon (sigmoid colectomy) **Low Resection:** Tumour in the upper rectum, more than 4 cm from anal verge
Abdominoperineal (AP) Resection	Low rectal tumour, < 4 cm from anal verge

The type of colectomies performed take into account the blood supply and lymphatic drainage of the bowel segment affected by the tumour. In general, the superior mesenteric artery and its branches supply to the right side of the colon and the proximal two thirds of the transverse colon. The left colon is supplied by the branches of the inferior mesenteric artery.

A Hartmann's procedure is usually reserved as an emergency procedure when an anastomosis is not feasible, such as in patients presenting acutely with either perforation secondary to diverticulitis or bowel obstruction secondary to a colorectal carcinoma. This involves resection of the rectosigmoid colon, with over-sewing of a rectal stump and fashioning a proximal end colostomy. The procedure is potentially reversible, although is associated with a high complication rate. It is rarely used as a palliative procedure in patients with colorectal carcinoma.

A stoma can be fashioned during bowel resection; for a discussion on stomas: (*see* Chapter 4, Abdominal stoma examination).

Case 5: Haematuria

Instructions: This man presents to the urology clinic with haematuria. Please take a focused clinical history.

Key features to look for:

- **Macroscopic or microscopic haematuria:** Ask the patient relevant questions to help you define whether the blood present in the urine is visible to the naked eye or has been detected on routine urine investigations, such as on a dipstick or in an MSU sample.
  - **Macroscopic:** This is when the patient can see blood in the urine, which is the most likely case in the exam. This is statistically more likely to be secondary to a malignant cause. Macroscopic haematuria is sometimes called frank or gross haematuria.

- ❑ **Blood clots:** Determine whether the patient can see clots in his or her urine; this is an indication for bladder irrigation via a three-way catheter due to the inherent risk of acute urinary retention when the clot blocks the urinary tract. Clots are usually from pathology high in the renal tract, such as from the pelvi-ureteric junction.
- – **Microscopic:** There are various arbitrarily defined limits to what is considered haematuria on dipstick or microscopy, and in some cases it can even be a normal finding. Malignancies, however, should always be excluded. Benign disease is statistically more likely, such as stones or glomerulonephritis, amongst others.

Authors' Top Tip

Distinguishing the causes of haematuria based on macroscopic or microscopic findings is difficult, as many aetiologies can present in either way. The important point to remember is that macroscopic haematuria is more likely to be a sign of malignancy.

Microscopic haematuria is the presence of >5 red blood cells per high power field on urine microscopy.

(Surgical Definition)

Authors' Top Tip

A woman who has her period will invariably have blood in her urinalysis. Do not attribute haematuria to contamination from periods until you have excluded urological causes.

- ■ **Presence of pain:** Whether the patient has pain associated with haematuria is a key distinguishing feature; pain generally implies an infective or inflammatory process, whereas painless haematuria typically occurs as a result of malignancy in the urinary tract.

Table 2.14: Causes of painful and painless haematuria

Presence of pain	Causes
Painless	**Cancer:** Until proved otherwise (most commonly transitional cell carcinoma of the bladder); TB.
Painful	**Dysuria (pain on urination):** Urethral stone, urethritis or trauma. **Suprapubic tenderness:** UTI, cystitis. **General abdominal pain:** Renal stones anywhere along the urinary tract. **Loin pain:** Pyelonephritis, stones, renal cell carcinoma. **Colicky:** Colicky pain that radiates from loin to groin is usually ureteric stones; clot colic.

> ## Authors' Top Tip
>
> *Bleeding from the renal tract, particularly at the renal pelvis itself, can cause colicky pain similar to ureteric stones as the clot passes down the ureters. This is called 'clot colic'. However, when you see patients in the emergency setting the most likely cause are calculi causing renal colic.*

- **Pattern:** The relationship of haematuria to the urinary stream can help determine the likely origin of bleeding.
  - **Total haematuria:** Blood throughout the stream suggests the presence of pathology in the upper urinary tract or bladder.
  - **Initial haematuria:** Blood at the start of the stream suggests bleeding from the urethra or the prostate.
  - **Terminal haematuria:** Blood at the end of the stream suggests pathology from the prostate or bladder (particularly the bladder neck).
- **Lower urinary tract symptoms (LUTS):** It is important to illicit symptoms that may be suggestive of underlying prostatic disease, such as benign prostatic hyperplasia (BPH), malignancy or UTI; all of which can cause haematuria.
  - **Storage symptoms:** These are typically seen in patients with distal ureteric or bladder stones, malignancy, infection, cystitis or bladder wall pathology, including fibrosis and oedema leading to a reduced functional capacity.
    - ❑ Elicit the symptoms of urinary frequency, urgency, dysuria and nocturia.
  - **Voiding symptoms:** Seen in those with urethral strictures or prostatic disease (benign or malignant), leading to bladder outflow obstruction (BOO).
    - ❑ Ask specifically for hesitancy, poor stream and terminal dribbling.

> ## Authors' Top Tip
>
> *LUTS used to be called symptoms of 'prostatism', which implied that the cause was prostatic in origin, which is not always true, so the term has been replaced with LUTS.*

- **Risk factor assessment:** Risk of urothelial cancers can be increased by:
  - **Cigarette smoking:** This increases the risk of renal cell carcinoma, TCC bladder and prostate cancer.
  - **Dye exposure:** Patients who have worked in factories with dyes, rubber or chemicals are at increased risk of TCC bladder due to the carcinogenic effects of the aromatic hydrocarbons found in these substances.

- – **Schistosomiasis infection:** Travel to certain areas of North Africa and the Middle East or swimming in fresh water increases the risk of schistosomiasis infection, which can cause TCC bladder or SCC bladder cancer due to chronic irritation.
- **Medications:**
  - – **Anticoagulants:** Ask if the patient is on any anticoagulants such as Warfarin, which can cause bleeding when the INR is high.
  - – **Others:** Some medications can cause urinary discolouration, which could be mistaken for haematuria such as rifampicin. The ingestion of certain foods such as beetroot can also lead to discolouration.
- **Medical history:** Ask specifically about:
  - – **Coagulopathy:** A history of coagulopathy in which the patient is prone to bleeding.
  - – **Sickle cell disease:** This causes renal infarction in a painful crisis.
  - – **Ureteric colic:** Previous episodes of intermittent loin pain suggest ureteric colic with small stones that may have passed spontaneously.
  - – **Renal biopsy:** Has the patient had a recent biopsy that could account for the haematuria?
  - – **Radiotherapy:** Haematuria post-radiotherapy occurs due to radiation-induced cystitis and urethritis, leading to episodic, self-limiting haematuria.
  - – **Transurethral resection of the prostate (TURP):** This can lead to minor bleeding postoperatively due to local trauma. Patients are often catheterised and have bladder irrigation to prevent the formation of a clot, which may lead to acute urinary retention. Occasionally the bleeding may be heavier and requires diathermy to control.
- **Family history:**
  - – Polycystic kidney disease (PCKD) is inherited in an AD fashion and is an important risk factor for renal cell carcinoma.
  - – Intrinsic renal disorders can be inherited and typically present with microscopic haematuria.
- **Associated symptoms:** These symptoms suggest either TB or malignancy:
  - – Metastatic spread causing weight loss or back pain.
  - – TB causing fever, night sweats and weight loss.

Completion

In actual clinical practice, it matters very little if haematuria is macroscopic or microscopic and whether it is terminal, throughout or at the beginning of the urinary stream, as haematuria is always considered abnormal and should always be investigated. However, for the purposes of your OSCE and the generation of a list of suitable differentials, it is important to illustrate that you are taking a complete and accurate history.

Authors' Top Tip

If a patient is on anticoagulants, you must investigate for another cause of haematuria. Never ignore patients with painless haematuria; they may have a transitional cell bladder carcinoma. There are dedicated one-stop haematuria clinics for this very purpose.

Viva questions

Q1   What are the causes of haematuria?

Table 2.15: Causes of haematuria

Cause	Aetiology
Medical	**Haematological:** Blood dyscrasia, liver disease **Drugs:** e.g. anticoagulants, Rifampicin, Metronidazole **Renal:** IgA nephropathy, glomerulonephritis, SLE, polycystic kidneys **Physiological:** Exercise induced **Others:** Post-radiotherapy, endocarditis, sickle cell, malaria
Surgical	**Kidney:** Stones, renal cell carcinoma, infection (TB, pyelonephritis), trauma **Ureters:** Stones, carcinoma **Bladder:** Stones, carcinoma, infection (TB, cystitis, schistosomiasis) **Prostate:** BPH, carcinoma **Urethra:** Stones, infection, carcinoma, trauma

Authors' Top Tip

Never forget, an elderly patient with a presumptive diagnosis of ureteric colic has a leaking AAA until proven otherwise.

Q2   How does a renal cell carcinoma classically present?
- As a triad of haematuria, an abdominal/loin mass and loin pain.

Renal cell carcinoma is the most common type of renal cancer and commonly referred to as Grawitz's tumour. A significant proportion of patients with renal cell carcinomas have an association with paraneoplastic syndromes, including hypercalcaemia, erythrocytosis and hypertension, amongst others.

A paraneoplastic syndrome is a collection of signs and symptoms due to a substance emanating from a tumour or as a consequence of the presence of that tumour. The condition occurs remotely from the tumour itself and is not due to the local presence of cancer cells, nor its metastases.

(Surgical Definition)

Q3   How would you investigate a patient with haematuria?
  ▪ USS KUB and flexible cystoscopy.

(Average Response)

The prevalence of malignancy in the urinary tract is significant, and so most investigations are aimed at ruling out renal tract carcinoma. All patients with haematuria should be referred to the one-stop haematuria clinic, where the following investigations are undertaken:

  ▪ **DRE:** Although this is traditionally part of your abdominal or pelvic clinical examination, the rectal exam is performed as an investigation in its own right. A craggy prostatic mass, nodules or loss of the normally palpable sulcus between the two lobes of the prostate suggests prostate cancer. BPH can also cause haematuria in which the prostate is large and vascular, so a smoothly enlarged prostate with symptoms of bladder outflow obstruction is likely to be due to this.
  ▪ **Urine sample:**
    – **Dipstick:** This is a useful screening test for a UTI, where leucocytes and nitrites will be positive; also used to look for microscopic blood that if identified in a patient presenting acutely with abdominal/loin pain should prompt consideration of renal stones. If protein is found, then this is highly suggestive of intrinsic renal causes, especially in children and young adults.
    – **MC&S:** Patients who complain of cystitis symptoms may have an underlying urine infection in which the causative organism can be identified on microscopy; red cell casts can also be seen, which suggest intrinsic renal disease. If crystals are found, this may suggest an underlying condition that increases the risk of renal calculi, e.g. calcium oxalate in calcium stones (the most common type of renal stones).
    – **Cytology:** To look for abnormal urothelial cells seen in cancer.
    – **TB:** Patients at high risk for TB may benefit from sending three early morning urine samples to rule out TB as a cause, especially in patients with an initial sterile pyuria.
  ▪ **Blood tests:**
    – **FBC:** To check for anaemia due to massive blood loss or anaemia of chronic disease due to malignancy.
    – **U&E:** These results may be deranged in cases of obstruction from a stone leading to acute renal failure.
    – **Clotting:** To check for a coagulopathy or in monitoring of patients on anticoagulants.
    – **PSA:** To be done in all male patients to exclude prostate carcinoma; be aware that a normal PSA (<4 ng/mL) does not rule out prostate carcinoma and that PSA increases with age.

Authors' Top Tip

It is important you take a blood test for PSA before the patient is catheterised, as instrumentation may lead to an inadvertent rise that may be mistaken for carcinoma.

The predictive value of PSA for prostate cancer increases when used in combination with DRE in patients being considered for prostate biopsy. However, PSA is not specific to prostate cancer and a raised PSA can be due to many causes

Table 2.16: PSA levels

PSA (ng/mL)	Causes
<4	Normal
<10	BPH, chronic prostatitis, ejaculation, DRE
>10	Prostate cancer, prostatitis, urinary retention/ catheterisation, TURP, prostate biopsy, UTI
>20	Prostate cancer, UTI, acute prostatitis, TURP, prostate biopsy

- ■ **Imaging:**
  - – **CXR:** This is a useful investigation in a patient suspected of having TB, or in a patient with renal cell carcinoma who has metastases, where classically multiple opacities are seen in the CXR; these are called 'cannonball metastases'.
  - – **IVU & KUB:** If the patient presents with ureteric colic, this can help identify the level of obstruction; 80% of renal stones are radio-opaque. However, this investigation is being phased out in favour of CT KUB, as its sensitivity is only 70–80% and has the added risk of using contrast material, which can lead to contrast-induced nephropathy.
  - – **Plain CT KUB:** This is now the first-line investigation for a patient presenting with renal calculi. This is a non-contrast scan that will determine the location, size and number of stones anywhere in the renal tract, as well as quantify the degree of hydronephrosis. It also helps identify other pathology that could mimic ureteric colic, such as a leaking AAA.
  - – **USS KUB:** Most patients have an USS of the renal tract to identify any obvious pathology, but with the advent of CT, this is becoming less popular. Furthermore, any patient found to have pathology on USS will have a CT scan eventually anyway. It is particularly good at differentiating between cysts and solid masses in the kidney, can estimate prostate size and is used for radiological guidance during interventional procedures such as percutaneous nephrostomy insertion in an infected hydronephrosis.
  - – **Flexible cystoscopy:** This is the gold standard investigation in haematuria and is used to image the bladder and biopsy any suspicious lesions; if there is a high suspicion of bladder cancer, then the patient may have a rigid cystoscopy and/or transurethral resection of the bladder tumour (TURBT) at the same sitting. Almost all patients with haematuria, even asymptomatic haematuria, are offered this investigation.
- ■ **Renal team referral:** Once malignancy and stones have been ruled out as possible causes, and if all results of the standard tests are normal, most patients are referred to Nephrology to look for intrinsic renal causes for the haematuria, such as glomerulonephritis.

(Good Response)

Authors' Top Tip

An elderly man with painless haematuria has transitional cell bladder carcinoma until proven otherwise.

Case 6: Dysphagia

Instructions: This 70-year-old gentleman presents with difficulty in swallowing. Please take a focused clinical history.

Key features to look for:
- **Assess dysphagia:**
  - **Absolute/partial:** Enquire as to the degree of dysphagia. Absolute dysphagia is when the patient is drooling saliva; this is typically seen in patients with epiglottitis when their airway is at risk of compromise; this is an emergency. Partial dysphagia is when the patient can swallow liquids or solids and is more representative of what you will see in the exam.
  - **Intermittent episodes:** Dysphagia can be intermittent when, for example, the stomach externally compresses the oesophagus in a paraoesophageal hiatus hernia; this is also seen in the early stages of achalasia.
  - **Localisation:** Patients who have a pharyngeal pouch can often localise the site of discomfort to an area just behind the manubrium; this is where the pouch is compressing the oesophagus. A female patient who complains of dysphagia at the upper third of the oesophagus is likely to have Plummer-Vinson syndrome, causing a post-cricoid web.
  - **Relation to solids/liquid:** The pattern of dysphagia and its progression can also be useful differentiating features.
    - **Solids progressing to liquids:** Dysphagia that was initially to solids and has progressed to liquids is highly suggestive of malignant disease and warrants urgent referral and investigation.
    - **Solids and liquids equally:** Achalasia typically causes dysphagia to liquids and solids in equal amounts; this is due to a failure of the LOS to relax.
  - **Duration of symptoms:**
    - **Sudden onset:** This could be due to caustic stricture formation after ingestion of corrosive materials; after the initial episode, a later stricture can occur several months afterwards.
    - **Period of days:** The cause is likely to be oral in origin, such as pharyngitis or tonsillitis.
    - **Acute onset:** A rapid onset over a period of a few weeks in an elderly male is likely to be oesophageal cancer.

- **Associated symptoms:**
  - **Neck lumps:** A man with a left-sided neck lump associated with dysphagia is likely to have a pharyngeal pouch.
  - **Halitosis:** This is typically seen in patients with a pharyngeal pouch due to stagnant decomposing food collecting in the pouch.
  - **Regurgitation:** On lying down, there may be regurgitation of food in a pharyngeal pouch with consequent coughing, and in some cases aspiration of contents into the lung. Occasionally when this is a recurrent affair it causes nocturnal asthma in the patient.
  - **Hiccups:** Irritation of the diaphragm can cause hiccups in those with a paraoesophageal hiatus hernia.
  - **Haemoptysis:** Patients who have an underlying bronchogenic carcinoma causing extrinsic compression of the oesophagus may present with haemoptysis.
- **Alarm symptoms:** Symptoms suggestive of malignancy include:
  - **Weight loss:** This is the second most common symptom after dysphagia, and can be dramatic (several stones in a period of a few weeks).
  - **Hoarse voice:** This occurs when there is involvement of the recurrent laryngeal nerve, which is a branch of the vagus nerve and implies a highly malignant tumour. This may manifest as a persistent bovine cough.
- **Cancer risk factor assessment:**
  - **Increased risk of adenocarcinoma:**
    - **Barrett's oesophagus:** This occurs secondary to prolonged reflux of stomach contents, leading to columnar metaplasia of the normal oesophageal stratified squamous non-keratinised epithelium. The metaplasia most commonly occurs in the distal third.
    - Patients often undergo surveillance to monitor this condition, and those with high-grade dysplasia or invasive adenocarcinoma are referred for surgical resection.
  - **Increased risk of squamous cell carcinoma:** This can occur anywhere along the length of the oesophagus. Risk factors include:
    - Tobacco smoking, high alcohol intake and a Western diet.
    - **Achalasia:** An oesophageal dysmotility disorder where the lower oesophageal sphincter (LOS) fails to relax.
    - **Oesophageal webs:** These lead to obstruction of the lumen, resulting in dysphagia. A well-known example is Plummer-Vinson Syndrome, where an oesophageal web is commonly seen in middle-aged women and is thought to occur secondary to iron deficiency anaemia. This web has the potential for malignant transformation.
    - **Oesophageal strictures:** These caustic strictures commonly occur if the patient has previously ingested corrosives either accidentally or intentionally.

- **Past medical history:** There are many medical conditions that can indirectly cause dysphagia, so it is important you ask specifically for the following:
  - **Neurological:** Recent stroke, myasthenia gravis, motor neurone disease, Guillain-Barre syndrome.
  - **Rheumatological:** Scleroderma, which can cause an oesophageal web.
  - **Cardiovascular:** Mitral stenosis, which leads to left atrial enlargement and can cause external compression of the oesophagus, as the two structures are closely related.
  - **Foreign body:** Usually the patient will offer this to you, but in children and mentally disabled patients you must always consider this. In elderly patients this may even be their false teeth!
  - **Gastro-oesophageal reflux:** Patients which chronic reflux disease can develop inflammatory strictures.
  - **Immunocompromised Patients:** Patients who are diabetic, on steroids or antibiotics, or are immunocompromised for any other reason are at increased risk of oral, pharyngeal and oesophageal fungal infections manifesting as candidiasis and viral infections, most commonly herpes and CMV.
  - **Radiation exposure:** Patients who may have had radiotherapy to the chest or mediastinum are at increased risk of developing a stricture due to irradiation.

Completion

It is important to take a focused history, as there are many causes of dysphagia. The key is to recognise alarm symptoms, which in conjunction with dysphagia would warrant urgent referral under the two-week-wait cancer route to rule out an upper GI cancer.

Upper GI endoscopy (OGD) is the diagnostic test of choice, and high-risk patients can be referred directly to the open-access endoscopy clinic for biopsy. The management is as for any cancer, i.e. that is with an MDT approach.

Dysphagia is difficulty in swallowing due to an inefficiency of the normal physiology of swallowing to take place, whereas odynophagia is pain on swallowing.

(Surgical Definition)

Authors' Top Tip

Do not confuse the term with dysphasia, which means difficulty in speech.

Table 2.17: Motility disorders causing dysphagia

Variable	Pharyngeal pouch	Diffuse oesophageal spasm	Achalasia
Age	Elderly	Middle age	Middle age
Aetiology	Pulsion diverticulum of the pharynx through Killian's dehiscence	Spasm of the oesophagus	Unknown, but most likely due to the degeneration of Auerbach's plexus, leading to failure of LOS to relax
Clinical features	Dysphagia and left-sided neck lump that gurgles on palpation (Boyce's sign); halitosis and regurgitation of food	Angina-like pain	Dysphagia for solids and liquids equally
Investigations	Barium swallow demonstrates pouch	Corkscrew appearance on Barium swallow; nutcracker oesophagus on manometry	'Bird's beak' appearance on barium swallow; increased pressures on manometry
Management	Surgical excision	Conservative, Nifedipine	Balloon dilatation, Botulinum toxin injection, Heller's cardiomyotomy

---

Authors' Top Tip

Pharyngeal pouch is one of the few causes of dysphagia that is a known contraindication to OGD due to the risk of perforation. And so the best first-line investigation is a contrast swallow, not an OGD.

Viva questions

Q1 What are the causes of dysphagia?
- Common causes of dysphagia include: stroke, motor neurone disease, pharyngeal pouch and oesophageal cancer.

(Average Response)

- The causes of dysphagia can be divided into neurological and non-neurological causes.
- **Neurological causes include:** stroke (most common), bulbar palsy, myasthenia gravis, etc.

- **Non-neurological causes can be divided into:** mechanical and non-mechanical causes.
- **Non-mechanical causes include:**
  - **Within the mouth:** oral candidiasis, oral carcinoma, epiglottitis, tonsillitis, oesophagitis, aphthous ulcers.
  - **Within the pharynx:** pharyngitis, pharyngeal pouch, retropharyngeal abscess.
- **Mechanical causes:** can be classified into causes within the lumen, outside the lumen and in the wall:

Table 2.18: Mechanical causes of dysphagia

Mechanical	Cause
In the lumen	Food bolus, foreign body, oesophageal web (due to, e.g. Plummer-Vinson syndrome, scleroderma).
In the wall	**A benign stricture:** due to trauma – which can be accidental or iatrogenic (e.g. endoscopy); chronic oesophagitis – which can be due to ingestion of corrosive liquids. **A malignant stricture:** due to carcinoma. **Dysmotility disorders:** achalasia, diffuse oesophageal spasm. **Others:** oesophageal carcinoma.
Outside the lumen	Bronchogenic carcinoma, mediastinal lymphadenopathy and lymphoma, retrosternal goitre and thyroid cancer, thoracic aortic aneurysm, left atrial hypertrophy, paraoesophageal hiatus hernia.

(Honours Response)

Q2 What is achalasia?

(Difficult Question)

- This is a dysmotility disorder characterised by the inability of the lower oesophageal sphincter (LOS) to relax, with absence of peristalsis.
- This is most likely due to the degeneration of Auerbach's plexus.
- This condition is clinically indistinguishable from Chaga's disease, which is a parasitic infection with *Trypanasoma cruzi*; endemic in Brazil.
- Achalasia is associated with an increased risk of oesophageal cancer (specifically squamous cell carcinoma).
- Barium swallow classically demonstrates the 'bird's beak' appearance.

Auerbach's plexus is one of the nerve plexi responsible for mediating neural control of the GI system through which food movement and its digestion are coordinated. It is found between the circular and longitudinal smooth muscle layers of the GI tract wall.

Q3 How would you differentiate between achalasia and oesophageal carcinoma on imaging, excluding CT Scans?

(Honours Question)

- Oesophageal carcinoma characteristically shows a stricture (similar to the apple core lesion in the bowel), which is sometimes described as giving a 'shouldered' appearance on barium swallow.

- The most common differential diagnosis on imaging is achalasia, which can look very similar on a contrast study, although it has a characteristic 'bird's beak' (or 'rat's tail') appearance.
- To differentiate on barium swallow, the size of the proximally dilated oesophagus is taken into account.
- With oesophageal cancer, progression is so rapid that the **dilatation is less** than with achalasia.
- Also, the consequent dilatation seen on barium swallow in achalasia affects the distal third, whereas oesophageal cancer can affect any third of the oesophagus (although most commonly this is also the distal third due to an increasing incidence of Barrett's oesophagus).
- Furthermore, in achalasia there is **absence of the gastric air bubble** on a plain film chest X-ray, whereas with oesophageal cancer there is not.

For contrast images: (*see* Chapter 12, Case 2).

Q4   Do you know of any regions within the oesophagus of natural constriction?

(Honours Question)

- There are several anatomical areas of constriction in the oesophagus. These are important to be aware of when, e.g. passing an endoscope, so as to avoid iatrogenic perforation; foreign bodies may also lodge there, and these sites are also common areas for the development of strictures and carcinoma.
- There are four areas; from proximal to distal:
  - The cricopharyngeal sphincter.
  - The aortic arch.
  - The left main bronchus.
  - The diaphragm.

The oesophagus is a 25-cm-long, hollow muscular tube that extends from the cricoid cartilage at the level of C6 to the gastro-oesophageal junction at the level of T10. The oesophagus passes through the right crus of the diaphragm at the level of T8 and enters the cardia of the stomach 2–3 cm distal to this.

Authors' Top Tip

If you ever get a patient who has just had an OGD present acutely with searing chest pain, iatrogenic oesophageal perforation will be the most likely cause.

CHAPTER 3

Skin and surgical scars

3.1 SKIN CANCERS

The skin is the largest and most vulnerable organ of the body. It is involved in a number of important jobs; these include providing a protective surface for the contents of the body, helping with thermoregulation, sensation and the storage of vitamin D, water and fat. It is made up of a number of layers, each of which has its own functions.

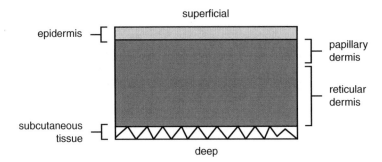

Figure 3.1: Skin layers

Within the field of surgery you are often presented with a skin lesion that has been referred for excision or an excision biopsy, so it is important you know what you are presented with before you excise the lesion. Accurate diagnosis starts with a good history, and although the examination is of primary importance here, histology will confirm your diagnosis. Of course in finals, you will have to work without histology and therefore should be able to come up with a reasonable list of differential diagnoses of any skin lesion presented to you. Even if you are unsure of the diagnosis, being able to examine and describe the lesion competently will have scored you most, if not all of the marks.

In some cases, the examiner may give you the opportunity to take a brief history; usually this is in the form of the examiner saying 'Would you like to ask the patient any questions?' Remember to keep your questions focused; you will not have time to take a full history. Features in the history of particular interest with skin lesions are:

- **Duration:** The length of time the lesion has been present for.
- **Changing lesion:** Have the lesion(s) changed, increased or decreased in size, disappeared then reappeared? If this is the case how many times has this happened, and is there any relationship to the season? Or any other identifying features, e.g. bleeding, itching?
- **Inheritance:** Family history of the condition.
- **Environmental influence:** Occupation and hobbies; e.g. does the patient spend a significant time out in the sun? Does he or she use sun beds frequently?
- **Drug side effect:** Is the patient taking any medications?
- **Hypersensitivity:** Any known allergies?
- **Patient history:** Has he or she had anything like this before, and if so how was it treated?

When examining a lesion the same basic principles apply as to any other systems exam. There is an emphasis on general inspection of the body surface first before moving on to a more focused assessment of the lesion identified. In actual clinical practice it is important to ask patients to remove any make-up, as this may distort the lesion. There are various associated features that you could look for on systems examination as part of your skin lesion examination; however, as the emphasis is on surgical finals, we suggest you refer to a good dermatology textbook because this will be an invaluable resource for your medical finals.

Clinical examination

Introduction
As for any clinical encounter (*see* Chapter 1, Section 1.3).

Inspection
✔ Describe general characteristics of lesion
- **Site:** The site will help you in part to decide the possible diagnoses; e.g. is the lesion on a sun-exposed area, raising the possibility of a malignancy, or present on the palms and soles? Is there a special predilection for the flexor or extensor surfaces or is there sparing of certain areas?
- **Distribution:** Is it symmetrical (e.g. psoriasis, vitiligo) or asymmetrical? On sun-exposed areas only?
- **Size:** If a discrete lesion, estimate the size in centimetres.
- **Shape/surface appearance:** Whether round, oval or irregular.
- **Number:** Comment on the number of lesions present; is there a single lesion or multiple lesions? Or is the appearance more suggestive of a rash?
- **Extent of involvement:** Is the lesion localised, regionalised or is there widespread involvement? Is it disseminated?

- **Arrangement:** Comment also on the arrangement of the lesion, i.e. discrete, grouped, annular or linear.
- **Colour:** Describe colour of the overlying skin. Is it one discrete colour or is it variegated?

Table 3.1: Overlying skin colour

Colour	Possible pathology
Hypopigmentation/paler skin	Loss of melanocytes
Red	Erythema – localised inflammation or infection
Yellow	Jaundice, xanthoma, xanthelasma
Orange	Hypercarotenemia – a benign condition following excess dietary intake of beta-carotene (a vitamin A precursor) found in orange/yellow vegetables and fruits. The skin discolouration is most obvious on the palms and soles
Purple	Kaposi's sarcoma and haemangioma; if violaceous, suggestive of lichen planus
Purple/grey	Ischaemic skin
Tanned	Haemochromatosis
Bluish or silverfish tinge to skin	Secondary to drug deposition, e.g. associated with amiodarone, minocycline
Black	Seen with melanocytic skin lesions such as a naevi or melanoma. Also seen in infarcted skin or gangrene caused by arterial insufficiency.
Blue	Mongolian spot/blue naevus
Discoloured fingernails	Green fingernails: infection by *Pseudomonas aeruginosa.* White fingernails: hypoalbuminemia, hereditary

Palpation

✔ Describe the texture
- This may be palpable or visible and helps in the diagnosis of the lesion, e.g. in lichenification, where there is thickening of the skin following repeated rubbing, and the skin markings become more obvious.
- Is the surface smooth, scaly, crusty or rough? Can you remove the crust or scales?
- On deeper palpation using the pulps of your thumb and index finger, is the lesion soft, firm or hard?

Lesion primary morphology

✔ Describe characteristic morphology
- This describes the physical changes in the skin and helps you to describe the type of lesion.

Table 3.2: Common lesions

Lesion	Morphology
Macules	Non-palpable lesions; usually <10 mm in diameter, represented by a colour change on the skin, e.g. a freckle. If >10 mm in diameter, then referred to as a patch.
Papules	This is also <10 mm in diameter, but this lesion is solid and palpable with distinct borders, e.g. a naevus, seborrhoeic and actinic keratosis.
Plaques	Palpable lesions that are raised or depressed compared to the skin surface; these are >10 mm in diameter, e.g. the plaque of psoriasis.
Nodules	Solid, raised lesion >10 mm in diameter and extends to the dermis or subcutaneous tissue, e.g. lipoma, BCC.
Vesicles	These are clear, fluid filled lesions measuring <10 mm in diameter. Seen in dermatitis herpetiformis.
Bullae	Clear, fluid-filled blisters that are >10 mm in diameter, e.g. seen following bites or burns and in pemphigus vulgaris and bullous pemphigoid.
Pustules	Inflamed vesicles containing pus seen in bacterial infections, folliculitis; larger lesions are known as an abscess.
Petechiae	Small, non-blanching areas of haemorrhage in the skin, e.g. seen in vasculitis and meningitis.
Purpura	This is a larger area of haemorrhage that may be palpable. Also known as ecchymosis or bruises.
Urticaria (wheals/ hives)	This appears as pink, raised lesions secondary to localised oedema and can occur following hypersensitivity drug reactions, a reaction to temperature or sunlight, or following local pressure. This lesion is normally transient, lasting less than 24 hours.
Ulcers	Here some or all of the dermis is lost, including the epidermis (*see* Chapter 9, Ulcers).
Erosions	This is an area of skin that has lost its epidermal layer; seen commonly after trauma.
Tumours	Solid mass of either the skin or subcutaneous tissue.
Scars	Areas of the skin that have undergone fibrosis as a result of injury. This can sometimes become thickened and enlarged. For instance, a keloid scar is seen when the original scar has hypertrophied and extended beyond the initial scar margin.

Lesion secondary morphology

✔ **Comment on lesion profile**
- Is it flat-topped, dome-shaped, pedunculated, etc.?

✔ **Describe surface features**
- Is there surface loss, i.e. loss of epidermis/dermis leading to erosions, ulcers or fissures?
- Is there presence of an exudate on the lesion, e.g. blood or pus?
- Is there crust on the surface where the exudate has dried up?

Complete the examination

Table 3.3: Common lesions in surgical practice

Lesion	Clinical features
Seborrhoeic keratosis (Seborrhoeic wart/ senile wart/ basal cell papilloma)	**Clinical presentation:** Benign condition seen in middle age and elderly populations. **Morphology:** Waxy pink papules in fair skinned people; waxy black/brown papules in darker skinned people. Can appear similar to cutaneous horn/wart secondary to epidermal hyperplasia. Lesion can appear pedunculated and often has a greasy appearance. There can be solitary or multiple growths. Notably they have distinct borders and are palpable elevated lesions, which help differentiate them from malignant lesions. However, if a lesion appears suddenly in clusters associated with pruritus, this may be secondary to an internal malignancy. **Special features:** Present in areas that contain a high number of sebaceous glands, i.e. the face, shoulder, chest and back. Rarely malignancy such as Bowen's disease can occur within seborrhoeic keratoses. When suspected an excision biopsy is required. **Treatment:** Managed conservatively with close patient monitoring. Can treat by curettage and cryoablation. May be surgically excised for cosmesis or excessive pruritus/pain.
Cutaneous horn	**Clinical presentation:** Usually benign; although in approximately 20% of cases malignancy is found at the base (most commonly an SCC). **Special features:** Common in the 60–70 age groups. Most common in light-skinned people. **Morphology:** Consists of a conical projection of keratin representing a horn. **Treatment:** Excision biopsy is recommended because of the risk of malignancy.

Table 3.4: Pre-malignant lesions

Lesion	Clinical features
Keratoacanthoma (Molluscum sebaceum)	**Clinical presentation:** Rapidly growing lesion (over 1–2 weeks) reaching 1–2 cm in size. It is a self-healing skin tumour. It grows far more rapidly than a skin cancer, hence the importance of identifying it within the history. **Morphology:** Dome-shaped, central keratin plug. **Epidemiology:** Ratio 3–4:1 (M:F); associated with sun exposure **Special features:** When present on sun-exposed areas in association with actinic keratosis it is called an actinic keratoachanthoma, which may actually be a well-differentiated SCC. Consider this if the lesion continues to grow, whereas normally it should involute, in which case ensure you assess for regional lymph nodes secondary to metastatic spread. **Treatment:** In most cases it is self limiting. Surgery is required for cosmesis and histology for suspicious features. Options: Surgical excision, curettage and electrodessication.

Table 3.4 Pre-malignant lesions (*Continued*)

Lesion	Clinical features
Actinic keratosis (Solar keratosis/senile keratoses)	**Clinical presentation:** Typically occurs in immunosuppressed patients such as those on immunosuppressive therapy following organ transplants. Unfortunately in these individuals there is a high risk of malignant transformation to SCC. **Morphology:** Scaly, rough, erythematous papules or plaques arising on sun-exposed areas. May be confused with a BCC due to its pigmented appearance in some cases. **Epidemiology:** Mainly in those over 50 years of age; M>F **Special features:** Has potential for malignant transformation to SCC. UV radiation is thought to be the most common cause for this lesion. Seen in fair-skinned people who have a history of chronic exposure to the sun. As such, patients whose professions involve prolonged time outdoors such as builders, farmers or those living in sunny climates are at risk. **Treatment:** Mainstay of treatment is prevention, best achieved with the aid of sunscreen to prevent further damage and reduce the risk of malignant transformation. Individual lesions can be treated by cryoablation, curettage or electrodessication. If there are multiple lesions, then treatment with 5–FU (fluorouracil) may be used. If the lesion appears suspicious, then a full-thickness biopsy is recommended.
Bowen's disease (Carcinoma in situ/squamous intraepidermoid neoplasia)	**Clinical presentation:** Classically occurs on sun-exposed skin but can also occur on non-sun-exposed skin, e.g. genitalia. **Morphology:** Lesions are scaly, pruritic, crusted or erythematous plaques. When a lesion with a similar morphology and histology is found in sun-exposed areas it is called an actinic keratosis. **Special features:** It is thought to be a carcinoma in situ, the margins of which do not extend beyond the dermal-epidermal junction. At some point, however, approximately 10% can become invasive. **Treatment:** Surgical excision is the recommended treatment of choice, although curettage, electrodessication, cryoablation and irradiation have also been used despite being associated with a high risk of recurrence.

Viva questions

Q1   What is the difference between a keloid and a hypertrophic scar?

(Difficult Question)

- These are lesions that occur secondary to an exaggerated tissue response during the healing process, leading to excessive fibrous tissue deposition. Both also appear in wounds.

Table 3.5: Keloid and hypertrophic scars

Clinical features	Keloid	Hypertrophic
Relationship to wound edge	Extends beyond the margins	Confined to the wound margins
Onset	Occurs several months after injury	Occurs soon after injury
Epidemiology	More common in Afro Caribbeans	Common in children
Special features	Can be tender or itchy	Commonly seen in burns
Recurrence post excision	Usually recurs	Does not recur

Case 1: Basal cell carcinoma (BCC)

Instructions: Please examine this lesion.

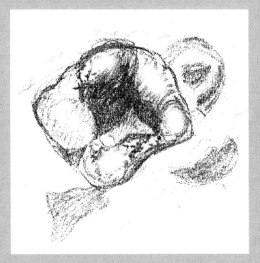

Figure 3.2: BCC

Key features to look for:
- Well-defined, non-tender nodular lesion in a sun-exposed area, e.g. face.
- With a rolled (not everted) pearly edge with central ulceration.
- There are some visible telangiectasia.
- The lesion is not fixed deeply (sign of invasion).

Complete the examination
✔ **Further examination**
- *'To complete my exam I would like to examine the regional lymphatic chains'.*

Your main differential diagnosis would be a malignant squamous cell carcinoma and a keratoacanthoma.

✔ Thank the patient
✔ Wash your hands
✔ Present your findings

This is the most common form of cutaneous cancer and accounts for 75% of skin cancers in the United Kingdom. There is a predilection for fair-skinned people, in those aged >50 years and in males. These cancer types occur in sun-exposed areas from the basal cells in the epidermis and are slow growing.

Although basal cell carcinomas rarely metastasise, they can become locally aggressive. Untreated they will continue to grow, eventually becoming an ulcer (rodent ulcer) and invade through the deeper layers of the tissue, eventually reaching the bone. Local recurrence is an issue after treatment.

Viva questions

Q1   What are the features of squamous cell carcinoma (SCC)?

(Difficult Question)

- SCC is the second most common non-melanoma skin cancer (NMSC) after BCC, occurring from the squamous cells in the epidermis.
- **Risk factors:** Incidence increases with increasing age (especially >70 years) and is more common in males.
- **Clinical features:** Occurs on sun-exposed areas and is slow growing. It usually metastasises to the surrounding structures, with distant metastases a rare occurrence.
- **Morphology:** Appears as a scaly lesion with an erythematous base or as a firm red papule. The lesion fails to heal and may bleed easily.
- **Special features:** SCC in situ is also known as Bowen's disease. It appears as large erythematous or brown plaques that are slightly raised with scaling on the surface. The SCC that is associated with Bowen's disease metastasises in as many as 33% of cases.

Q2   What are the treatment options for BCC and SCC?

(Honours Question)

- Treatment for both BCC and SCC requires an MDT approach, but typically involves:
    - Excision of the lesion with a pre-defined margin of clearance.
    - Usage of topical 5–FU or curettage and electrocautery if the lesion is small.
    - Radiotherapy if the lesion is too large for surgical excision or if operative management will be associated with disfiguration.
    - Radiotherapy following surgical excision to minimise recurrence risk.
    - Chemotherapy if metastases present.

Case 2: Malignant melanoma

Instructions: Please examine this lesion.

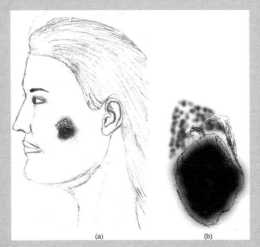

(a)   (b)

Figure 3.3a, b: Melanoma

Key features to look for:
- There is an *x*-centimetre, non-tender lesion on the left side of the face.
- It is ovoid in shape, appears raised and has an irregular outline.
- The lesion is black in colour with a nodular outline.
- There also appears to be some superficial spread that is variegated in colour.

Complete the examination
✔ Further examination
- *'To complete my exam I would like to examine the regional lymphatic chains, the liver and listen to the chest'.*

✔ Thank the patient
✔ Wash your hands
✔ Present your findings

Summarise as above and then say:
- *'I am concerned that this may be a suspicious lesion and I would like to exclude malignant melanoma'.*

Melanoma is a form of skin cancer with an annual incidence of >10 000 people in the United Kingdom. Over the past 10 years, incidence has doubled in the United Kingdom and has become the most common cancer in those aged 15–34 years (although it is more common in the older age group). It is frequently seen in fair-skinned people as a result of increased growth of melanocytes in the epidermis. It can occur as a dark macule/papule in a pre-existing naevi in half of all cases;

typically in women, this is seen on the legs; and in men, on the chest or back. This is more progressive than NMSC and will metastasise, making it the commonest cause of death from skin disease. Diagnosis involves excision biopsy and in some cases a sentinel node biopsy is also performed.

Authors' Top Tip

Always consider malignant melanoma if there has been a change in shape, size, colour or contour of a pre-existing lesion. A useful hint is in comparing this lesion to others present on the skin, there will be significant differences.

Viva questions

Q1 What are the different types of melanoma?

(Difficult Question)

■ There are several different types of melanoma.

Table 3.6: Types of melanoma

Type	Features
Superficial spreading	Most common (65%) form, occurs on any body site, looks like a flat, irregularly shaped and coloured lesion.
Nodular melanoma	Twenty per cent of cases and is polypoid in shape; colour can range from dark black/blue to blue/red to normal skin colour.
Lentigo maligna	Appears on sun-damaged areas, such as the face; more common in elderly where it appears as large areas of tan with brown in them; this becomes invasive in almost half the individuals affected by it.
Acral lentiginous	An uncommon form; occurs on the palms, soles and nail base; common in Africans.
Amelanotic	A rare form where the lesion is not pigmented; patients often present with metastatic spread to the lymph nodes and consequently have a poor prognosis.

■ The characteristic clinical examination features of melanoma can be remembered using the mnemonic ABCDE:
  – A: asymmetry.
  – B: border (irregular).
  – C: colour change, variation within single lesion (variegation).
  – D: diameter is usually >6 mm.
  – E: evolving, i.e. the lesion changes and eventually ulcerates and is more liable to bleed.

Q2 Do you know of any pathological staging systems for malignant melanoma?

(Honours Question)

- There are two commonly used: Clark's Levels and Breslow's Thickness; a combination of the two increases prognostic accuracy.
- Both assess depth of tumour invasion with respect to the epidermis.

Clark's Levels

- **Level I:** Invasion into epidermis only.
- **Level II:** Invades papillary dermis.
- **Level III:** Fills papillary dermis but doesn't invade reticular dermis.
- **Level IV:** Invades reticular dermis.
- **Level V:** Invades subcutaneous tissues.

Breslow's Thickness

Tumour invasion thickness versus approximate 10-year survival rates:
- **Thickness <0.76 mm:** Survival >90%.
- **Thickness >3 mm:** Survival ~50%.
- **Thickness >4 mm:** Survival <30%.

Q3   What features are associated with a poor outcome?

(Honours Question)

- A poor prognostic grade (*see above*).
- Ulceration; the presence of satellite lesions.
- Amelanotic melanoma and depigmentation.
- Male gender.
- A high mitotic index with aneuploidy.

3.2   SURGICAL SCARS

Although this is unlikely to be an OSCE station in its own right, students may be asked in an abdominal examination station what the name of a particular scar is and what they think the underlying operation was. We find many students struggle on this unnecessarily; therefore, we provide you with an outline of the most common scars you are likely to come across in finals and how to approach them in a logical manner.

Clinical examination

✔ **Identify scar**
- Name scars with their common eponymous names, if possible.
- If you do not know the names, then describe the scars anatomically, e.g. a 2-cm scar in the right groin.
- Comment on whether the scar appears recent or old.
  - **Recent:** Scar is usually raised and pink/red.
  - **Old:** By six months it is normally flat and the same colour as the surrounding skin.
✔ **Check for an incisional hernia**
- Ask patient to cough or raise head off the bed.
✔ **Suggest possible operations**
- The examiner may ask you to suggest some possibilities.

Authors' Top Tip

Even if you have no idea what the possible operation may be, do not panic. Use your understanding of the underlying organs in the region of the scar and you may be able to think of some possibilities. We have seen some candidates say that they do not know what the operation is but have made a logical 'guess', e.g. saying that there may have been an operation involving the bladder. At least this shows you are thinking rather than giving up and saying you do not know.

Case 1: Abdominal wall scars

Instructions: Please describe the surgical scars on this abdomen.

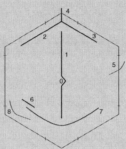

Figure 3.4: Abdominal scars

Table 3.7: Abdominal scars

Key	Scar name	Possible operation
1	**Midline laparatomy scar**	Exploratory laparotomy, hemicolectomy, Hartmann's, AAA repair **Upper midline scar:** Splenectomy (massive) **Lower midline scar:** Para-umbilical hernia repair, colectomy
2	**Kocher's or right subcostal**	Open cholecystectomy, partial liver resection, any biliary surgery
3	**Reversed Kocher's**	Open splenectomy
2+3	**Double Kocher's or rooftop scar**	Ivor Lewis (oesophagectomy), complex pancreatic/gastric surgery
2 3+4	**Mercedes scar or extended rooftop**	Complex upper-GI surgery, e.g. McKeown oesophagectomy, gastrectomy
5	**Left nephrectomy scar or loin incision**	Nephrectomy, specialist renal surgery
6	**Gridiron or McBurney's**	Appendicectomy
7	**Pfannenstiel**	**Pelvic surgery:** Bladder resection, prostatectomy, bilateral hernia repairs **Gynaecological:** Caesarean section, cystectomy, hysterectomy
8	**Rutherford Morrison or hockey stick**	Renal transplant

Authors' Top Tip

If you see a renal transplant scar, you can earn brownie points by telling the examiner you would look for its associated scars, e.g. AV fistula at the wrist, median sternotomy scar, CAPD (Tenckhoff) scar on abdominal wall or infraclavicular scars from previous dialysis access (Vas Cath insertions).

Completion

The gridiron scar for a classical approach for an appendicectomy is made as an incisional line perpendicular to McBurney's line at McBurney's point. McBurney's line is an imaginary line between the ASIS and the umbilicus. McBurney's point is one third of the distance from the ASIS to the umbilicus along McBurney's line.

Increasingly the transverse muscle splitting incision (Lanz) is being used for appendicectomy, as the cosmetic result is much better. This is because the incision follows Langers' lines.

Viva questions

Q1 What structures would you go through in an appendicectomy scar?

(Difficult Question)

From superficial to deep:
- Skin, subcutaneous tissue.
- Scarpa's fascia, linea alba.
- Muscle layers: external oblique, internal oblique then transversus abdominis.
- Transversalis fascia.
- Extra peritoneal fat then parietal peritoneum.

Q2 What structures would you go through in a midline laparotomy scar?

(Difficult Question)

From superficial to deep:
- Skin, subcutaneous tissue.
- Scarpa's fascia, linea alba.
- Transversalis fascia.
- Extra peritoneal fat then parietal peritoneum.

Q3 What are the advantages and disadvantages of the midline laparotomy scar?

(Honours Question)

Advantages
- Provides good access.
- Can be easily extended.
- Speed of closure and opening.
- Relatively avascular (linea alba).

Disadvantages

- Incision is more painful than transverse incision.
- Scar crosses Langer's lines, i.e. poor cosmetic appearance.
- Narrow linea alba below umbilicus; therefore, it can damage the bladder.

Case 2: Laparoscopic abdominal wall scars (Difficult Case)

Instructions: Please describe the surgical scars on this abdomen.

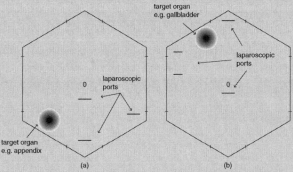

Figure 3.5: (a) Laparoscopic appendicectomy; (b) Laparoscopic cholecystectomy

Completion

Laparoscopic scars are difficult to see by their very nature, but increasingly laparoscopic surgery is becoming commonplace. It is important to bear in mind that even though there may be smaller individual scars in terms of size, collectively they may equal or even be greater than the original size of a single open-access incision.

Authors' Top Tip

If you see a tiny, barely visible scar around the umbilicus, this is likely to be a laparoscopic scar, usually for the insertion of the camera port.

Viva questions

Q1 Do you know what features determine the placement of laparoscopic ports?

(Honours Question)

- In general, ports should be placed away from areas of high risk, such as:
  - Previous scars, adhesions and known organomegaly.
  - The vessels of the anterior abdominal wall should be avoided, particularly the inferior epigastric artery.
- The minimum number of ports possible should used; typically three ports.

- The positioning of these three ports should then allow for the target organ to be at the apex of an imaginary diamond formed by the various ports as well as the target organ itself.
- The 10-mm port is for the camera and is useful for the removal of organs such as the gallbladder in a cholecystectomy. All other ports are typically 5 mm in size.

Q2 What are the advantages and disadvantages of laparoscopic surgery?

Table 3.8: Laparoscopic surgery

Variable	Description
Advantages	■ Shorter hospital stay and rehabilitation. ■ Less post-operative pain. ■ Better cosmetic result. ■ Less wound complications. ■ Decreased handling of organs, e.g. bowel. ■ Less trauma to tissues. ■ Later reduced incidence of post-operative adhesions.
Disadvantages	■ Lack of tactile feedback to the operating surgeon. ■ Longer operation times. ■ More technical expertise required, prolonged training. ■ Expensive equipment. ■ Difficulty in controlling massive bleeding. ■ Increased risk of iatrogenic injury to surrounding organs. ■ Not always feasible due to contraindications, e.g. adhesions.

CHAPTER 4

The surgical abdomen

4.1 EXAMINATION OF THE SURGICAL ABDOMEN

The examination of a surgical abdomen is very similar to the abdominal examination you have performed for medical finals, but with an emphasis on surgical causes.

It is best to think of the abdomen as being divided into four quadrants, or nine regions, as shown below:

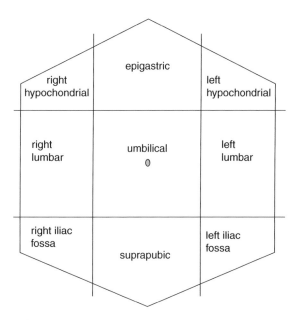

Figure 4.1: Abdominal regions

With this regional division in mind, think about the underlying organs in their respective region whenever you are examining a patient.

Table 4.1: Abdominal regions

Region	Underlying organ
Right hypochondrial	Liver, gallbladder, right kidney, hepatic flexure of colon
Right lumbar	Ascending colon, small bowel, right urinary tract
Right iliac	Caecum, appendix, terminal ileum, right ovary and right fallopian tube
Epigastric	Liver (left lobe), pylorus, duodenum, transverse colon, head and body of the pancreas
Umbilical	Duodenum, small bowel, abdominal aorta
Suprapubic	Bladder, uterus
Left hypochondrial	Spleen, stomach, splenic flexure of colon, tail of the pancreas, left kidney
Left lumbar	Descending colon, small bowel
Left iliac	Sigmoid colon, left ovary and left fallopian tube

With these two fundamental principles at the back of your mind, can you then examine a surgical abdomen competently. Below we describe a scheme you may wish to adopt when approaching the abdomen in surgical finals.

Clinical examination

Introduction
As for any clinical encounter: (*see* Chapter 1, Section 1.3). Specifically for this case:
- **Expose the patient adequately:** The patient needs to be exposed ideally from nipples to knees, but to maintain the patient's modesty, exposure from the xiphisternum to the pubis is adequate.
- **Position the patient appropriately:** The patient needs to be in a supine position, with the head resting on one pillow and arms by his or her sides; the level of the bed also needs to be at an appropriate height to make the examination comfortable for the examiner from a standing position.

Inspection
✔ Perform a general inspection from the end of the bed. Examine the following:
- **Paraphernalia:** Look around the bed for peripheral stigmata of disease. Is there a box to measure the patient's blood sugar? Is there a PCA or any other medications around?
- **Patient's demeanour:** Does the patient look comfortable? Or the patient look like he or she is in pain? A patient with peritonitis will classically lie very still, in contrast to the patient with some form of colic (renal, biliary, intestinal), who will be writhing in bed with spasmodic pain.

- **Degree of illness:** Does the patient look well or septic? Is he or she peripherally shut down; is there pallor or clamminess? In a peritonitic state, the patient will classically look pale with sunken eyes and have a greyish tinge to his or her face.
- **Any weight loss:** Is there evidence of weight loss or wasting? An individual considered to be cachectic (exhibiting severe weight loss) will normally have an underlying malignancy, although it can also be a feature of alcoholism or TB and is also seen in heart failure. Keep in mind that weight loss or wasting can also occur secondary to malabsorption.
- **Dehydration:** Does the patient appear to be dehydrated? Closer examination of the patient's skin turgor and mucous membranes will assist in deciding this.
- **Respiration:** Assess the respiratory rate and pattern – if the patient is peritonitic, he or she may take rapid, shallow breaths.
- **Any jaundice:** Does the patient look jaundiced? This is seen as a yellow discolouration to the skin and sclera resulting from an excess of bilirubin, which can be unconjugated or conjugated. Jaundice becomes clinically detectable at levels greater than 40 micromol/L; this may indicate liver disease or biliary tract obstruction.
- **Any skin changes:**
  - Look for purpura; which is an indication of impaired clotting.

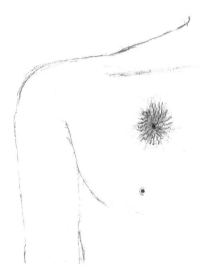

Figure 4.2: Spider naevi

  - Look for spider naevi. Greater than five above the nipple line in a superior vena caval distribution is pathognomonic of liver disease.
  - *Caput medusae* – these distended veins radiate away from the umbilicus secondary to severe portal hypertension. In obstruction of the inferior vena cava, blood flows superiorly in the dilated epigastric veins present on the abdominal wall.

✔ **Examine the hands**
  - **Temperature:** Feel for temperature; are they warm or cold and clammy?

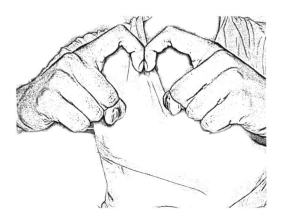

Figure 4.3: The diamond sign

  - **Nail changes:**
    – Digital clubbing – present in malabsorptive conditions, such as coeliac disease and IBD. Also present in cirrhosis. Clinically seen as a loss of the angle between the nail and the nail bed – the so-called diamond sign.
    – Koilonychia is present in iron deficiency anaemia.
    – Leukonchia – chronic liver disease.
  - **Hand abnormalities:**
    – Palmer erythema and Dupuytren's contracture – present in liver disease.
    – Pale skin creases – a sign of iron deficiency anaemia.
    – Pyoderma gangrenosum – present on the dorsum of the hand in inflammatory bowel disease.
  - **Tremor:** Examine for a flapping tremor; this is present in liver disease, particularly in encephalopathy. A similar tremor can also be seen in respiratory failure and electrolyte imbalance. To examine for this, ask the patient to extend the arms out in front and cock the wrists back, then look for movement.
  - **Assess the pulse:** Palpate the patient's pulse. Is he or she tachycardic? This is suggestive of pain, sepsis, dehydration or the presence of a fever. Ask the examiner for the patient's temperature.
✔ **Examine the face, neck and chest.**
  - **Eye signs:**
    – The Kayser Fleischer ring is present in Wilson's disease and appears around the cornea as a yellow/brown ring.
    – Pale conjunctiva is indicative of anaemia.
    – Look for evidence of jaundice in the sclera (ideally in natural daylight).
    – Look for xanthelasma, which appear as yellow plaques around the eyelids; these are seen in hypercholesterolaemia, primary biliary cirrhosis and in cases of biliary obstruction.

- **Mouth signs:** Look in the mouth for dry mucous membranes, furring of the tongue as seen in dehydration, aphthous ulcers in Crohn's disease, angular stomatitis in iron deficiency anaemia and an enlarged red beefy tongue as seen in anaemia. Note if the patient's breath smells ketotic (described as a sweet pear-like smell), or does the patient's breath smell of alcohol?
- **Assess for lymphadenopathy:** Briefly palpate for lymph nodes in the neck triangles, in particular palpate for the presence of a lymph node in the left supraclavicular fossa; when present this is known as Troisier's sign and is called a Virchow's node. This node drains the thoracic duct, which receives lymph drainage from the abdomen and the left side of the thorax. It is enlarged as a result of metastatic deposit from a malignancy anywhere in this region, although classically it is attributed to a gastric malignancy.
- **Chest wall signs:** Look for gynaecomastia and spider naevi in the superior vena caval distribution above the nipple line. Both are present in chronic liver disease.

✔ **Closer inspection of abdomen**

It is often useful to kneel down on the right side of the patient to the level of the patient's abdomen.

- **Abdominal contour:** Is it flat, scaphoid or distended?
  - **Scaphoid:** Seen in starvation, malnutrition.
  - **Distension:** Aetiology easiest remembered as the five F's: fluid, fat, flatus, faeces and foetus.
- **Scars:** Describe their location and the associated surgery, plus the characteristics of the scar, i.e. all scars are raised and red, but by 6 months they are normally flat and the same colour as the surrounding skin. If a scar becomes infected, it will appear to be more irregular than a normal scar that is healing by primary intention. Remember that scars have the potential to cause adhesions, which can cause intestinal obstruction. Laparoscopic scars may be difficult to see. Always check for an incisional hernia at this point (*see* Chapter 3, Surgical scars).
- **Abdominal wall hernia**: Describe its location; it could be a paraumbilical hernia or incisional hernia occurring at sites of old scars. Look for divarication of the recti; this is caused by weakening of the abdominal muscles, causing separation of the rectus abdominis muscles. This can be accentuated in the examination by asking the patient to lift his or her head off the couch and asking the patient to touch the chest wall with his or her chin, or by asking the patient to sit up.
- **Presence of stoma:** Describe its location, and start considering what type you think it may be, as very possibly you will be quizzed in the viva (*see* Abdominal stoma examination).
- **Skin changes:** Look for bruising, striae (which generally occur as a result of rupture of the reticular dermis); silver striae (which signify significant changes in weight); bluish striae (which are present in hypercortisolism) or prominent veins (these are present in obstruction of the portal venous system). Discolouration/ bruising present in a haemoperitoneum, secondary to haemorrhagic pancreatitis or ruptured ectopic pregnancy. Cullen's sign is bluish discolouration around the umbilicus; Grey Turner's sign is bluish discolouration at the flanks.

- **Abnormal movement:** Peristalsis (visible in intestinal obstruction), abdominal respiration (this is absent in peritonitis) or transmitted pulsation from the aorta in the epigastric region.
- **Masses:** These may be visible if they are large, in which case you should describe their location, shape and size.
- **Presence of drains:** You may see indwelling catheters, such as those used for peritoneal dialysis or for draining ascites.
- **Cough test:** Ask the patient to cough – this will be extremely painful in the presence of peritonitis, and the patient may even refuse to do this as a result.

Palpation

Always examine from the patient's right-hand side and kneel down to the patient's height. Before starting palpation of the abdomen, ask the patient to point to any site of pain and start away from this, working around the abdomen in a systematic manner. Whilst you are palpating, always look at the patient's face for signs of pain or discomfort.

✔ **Light and deep palpation**
- To palpate, use your four fingers, flexing at the MCPJ.
- Palpate systematically around the abdomen in all nine regions, beginning with light palpation, and then repeating the process with deeper palpation.
- On palpation, note:
  - **Soft/Hard:** If the abdomen is rigid all over and 'board-like' due to involuntary contraction of abdominal muscles, this is a strong indication of peritonitis. The patient will also be lying very still.
  - **Guarding:** This refers to tensing of the abdominal wall muscles as you apply pressure, in response to underlying peritoneal inflammation.
  - **Rebound tenderness:** This means that once you swiftly remove your palpating hand from the patient's abdomen, the patient experiences pain as the inflamed peritoneum is forced into contact with the underlying inflamed organ. A kinder way to examine for this is using percussion to illicit tenderness.

✔ **Palpate the liver**
- Place the dorsal edge of the index finger on the abdominal wall, starting at the right iliac fossa, and palpate deeply; if pain allows, gradually moving up towards the right hypochondrium, so you end up parallel to where you expect the liver edge to be.
- To feel for the liver edge, ask the patient to take in a deep breath whilst you are pressing inwards and upwards with your hand. As the patient is at maximal inspiration, ease the inward pressure; at this point you will feel the liver edge if it is palpable.
- The liver will normally be palpable just below the costal margin as it moves down a few centimetres on maximal inspiration. Follow the edge of the liver across the abdomen, working medially to the xiphisternum.

✔ **Palpate the spleen**
- This time working from the RIF towards the left hypochondrium and using the tips of your fingers, press inwards and upwards as the patient takes in a deep breath for you; work your way slowly up towards the left costal margin. In splenomegaly, you will feel the edge of the spleen before you reach this point.

- If this fails to illicit a palpable spleen, you can ask the patient to slowly roll onto the right-hand side and repeat the above procedure to accentuate any splenomegaly. You can place your other hand on the patient's ribcage on the left to offer support.
- In a normal individual, the spleen is not palpable. In pathological states, it increases in size and is thus palpable below the left costal margin.

✔ **Ballot the Kidneys**

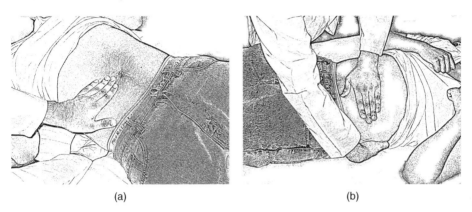

(a)   (b)

Figure 4.4a, b: Balloting

- Here you will be using two hands; beginning with the right loin, place one hand under the loin and use the other hand to palpate over the right lumbar region. Instruct the patient to take deep breaths in and out, and move your hands together to feel for an enlarged kidney, any kidney masses or tenderness in the loin. Now, repeat this on the other side with your hands in a comfortable position.
- Normally the lower pole of the right kidney is palpable; this is especially true in thin individuals. Enlargement of both kidneys is seen in polycystic kidney disease; unilateral enlargement may be seen in the presence of a tumour or hypertrophy.

✔ **Palpate other organs**
- Examine for an AAA (*see* Chapter 9, Section 9.1).
- **Focused visceral examination:** If necessary from the history, you can palpate for an enlarged bladder, or other palpable masses arising from the pelvis. Use the same method to palpate, but this time starting at the umbilicus and moving inferiorly to the symphysis pubis. If the patient is jaundiced, you may wish to palpate for a gallbladder, which if found is always pathological according to Courvoisier's Law.
- **Examine any masses:** Note that if any mass is palpable, it needs to be described in terms of its position, size, surface, consistency and all the factors that you would normally use to describe a lump, particularly whether the edge is palpable or whether the mass is associated with an enlarged palpable organ; you must note whether it is pulsatile or tender (*see* Chapter 5, Lumps and bumps).
- Interestingly, in cases of severe constipation you will be able to palpate faeces in the large bowel, most commonly in the sigmoid colon. You will know this is faeces, as there are usually multiple masses that are easily indentable on examination.

Percussion

■ This will allow you to determine the nature of any distension.
■ This is performed by placing your index finger flat on the abdominal surface horizontally and tapping the surface with the index finger of your other hand, listening for the sound it generates:
  – **Dull:** Solid or liquid underneath.
  – **Resonant:** Air.
■ You can also use percussion to demonstrate an enlarged intra-abdominal organ, such as an enlarged liver, spleen or bladder. Some candidates prefer to do this immediately after palpating each organ, rather than performing this as a separate routine.

Authors' Top Tip

We feel that eliciting peritonism using percussion is slightly kinder on a patient than using rebound tenderness.

✔ **Examine for ascites**

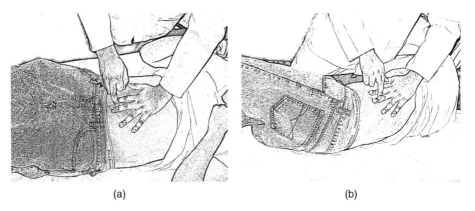

(a)   (b)

Figure 4.5a, b: Shifting dullness

If the history is suggestive of ascites or there is fullness at the flanks, you can demonstrate the presence of ascites by:
■ **Shifting dullness:** Percuss from the umbilicus laterally until there is a change in percussion note to dull; keep your finger at this point, and ask the patient to roll onto the opposite side, then wait for about 20 seconds to allow the fluid to displace to the other side. Start to percuss again, listening for a change in percussion note from dull to resonant. If the spot you marked now has a different percussion note, then this is positive for the presence of ascites. Repeat this by asking the patient to lie on his or her back again, and percuss back to the umbilicus, now towards the opposite flank.
■ **Fluid thrill:** This requires some experience. With the patient lying on his or her back, place your left hand on the patient's flank; using the right hand, flick at the right flank and feel for a fluid thrill/impulse at your left hand. This now needs to be repeated with the patient's hand placed in the midline of the abdomen, repeating the flick. Again repeat this on the opposite flank. The presence of a thrill is a positive sign.

> ### Authors' Top Tip
>
> *We suggest you use the shifting dullness technique in finals, as a fluid thrill is difficult to perform unless the patient has massive abdominal distension due to ascites.*

Auscultation

✔ Listen for bowel sounds
  - Peristalsis of the bowel results in gas and fluid being passed through the bowel lumen; this produces bowel sounds. In a normal state, these are heard as intermittent, low-pitched sounds. In pathological states, this changes.
  - Place the diaphragm of your stethoscope over the abdomen and listen for bowel sounds; this can be repeated in three different locations, and if no bowel sounds are heard, you must continue listening for at least 3 minutes to be confident of this.
    - **Absent sounds:** Paralytic ileus, peritonitis, obstruction, mesenteric ischaemia/infarction.
    - **Increased sounds:** Diarrhoea, obstruction.
    - **Tinkling:** Ileus, a later phase of obstruction.
✔ Listen for bruits
  - **Abdominal aorta:** Listen over the aorta for abdominal bruits caused by turbulent blood flow; your stethoscope needs to be placed above the level of the umbilicus as the aorta bifurcates at the level of L4, which is approximately at the level of the umbilicus. Bruits are best heard in the epigastric region.
  - **Renal artery:** Bruits may also be heard in renal artery stenosis, for which you place your stethoscope in the upper quadrants.
  - **Iliac/femoral artery:** To listen for bruits related to the iliac or femoral arteries, place your stethoscope in the lower quadrants; the presence of bruits here signifies the potential presence of peripheral vascular disease.

Special Tests

These tests are not done routinely but can be performed depending on your initial clinical diagnosis to either refute or confirm them.

Complete the examination

✔ Further examination
  - *'To complete my examination, I would like to perform a digital rectal examination, examine the external genitalia and the hernial orifices, perform a urine dipstick and send off an MSU, including a pregnancy test in females'.*

Some may argue that a full abdominal examination includes examination of the pelvis in the female; you can mention that you may consider this if the presentation is suggestive of possible pelvic pathology, in which case your history would extend to elicit symptoms related to this.

✔ Thank the patient
✔ Wash your hands
✔ Present your findings

Table 4.2: Special tests

Special test	Features
McBurney's point tenderness	This is regarded as being the site of maximal tenderness in cases of acute appendicitis; it is found one-third of the way from the ASIS to the umbilicus.
Psoas sign	Place your hand above the patient's right knee and apply resistance; next ask the patient to flex at the hip joint. If by doing this it causes increased abdominal pain, then the test is considered to be positive for appendicitis.
Obturator sign	Lift the patient's right leg with the knee flexed; internally rotate the hip joint stretching the obturator muscle; if this causes increased abdominal pain, again this is a positive sign for appendicitis.
Rovsing's sign	Palpate in the LIF; on releasing the pressure, if the patient experiences pain in the RIF, the test is considered to be positive for appendicitis.
Cough test	Pain experienced by the patient when asked to cough in peritonitis, as this moves the peritoneum and causes pain when there is peritoneal irritation. This is also another way to elicit rebound tenderness.
Carnett's sign	An eponymously named finding wherein cases of acute abdominal pain the pain can either increase or remain unchanged when asked to tense the muscles of the abdominal wall. This can be done by either asking the patient to lift the head and shoulders off the examining couch or to straight-leg raise both legs. If the pain is increased, then this is a positive finding and suggests that the pain is likely to be a result of abdominal wall pathology, such as a rectal sheath haematoma, as opposed to pain caused by intra-abdominal pathology.
Succussion splash	Present in gastric outflow obstruction from the distended stomach containing gas and fluid. Elicited by shaking patient with hands on either side of the ribcage.
Boas' sign	This is pain that radiates from an inflamed gallbladder in acute cholecystitis to the tip of the right scapula. This also leads an area of skin just below the scapula to become extremely sensitive to touch, resulting in pain (hyperaesthesia).

Some institutes teach that auscultation should be performed after inspection and before the rest of the examination. This is primarily due to the fact that by palpating and percussing over the abdomen you may artificially alter the activity of the bowel and hence the bowel sounds heard. In addition, if you cause the patient pain or discomfort earlier in the examination by assessing for rebound tenderness, by the time you get to auscultation the patient may not be so cooperative with you. We suggest you to follow the pattern taught at your particular medical school.

Viva questions

Q1 What are the causes of digital clubbing?
This is an absolute classical question, and although the most common cause is idiopathic, your answer needs to be classified to score the maximum marks available.

Table 4.3: Causes of clubbing

Classification	Causes
Gastrointestinal causes	Inflammatory bowel disease, primary biliary cirrhosis, coeliac disease
Respiratory causes	Bronchogenic carcinoma; suppurative lung disease, e.g. bronchiectasis; cystic fibrosis; mesothelioma, fibrosing alveolitis
Cardiac causes	Congenital cyanotic heart disease, endocarditis
Other causes	Familial, Graves' disease

There is an actual grading system to measure the relative degree of clubbing; the more ambitious student may wish to learn this. You would not be expected to understand the pathophysiology of clubbing. There is a standardised method for examining digital clubbing, which is better suited for medical finals.

Q2 What is the significance of palpating a tender gallbladder?

(Difficult Question)

- This elicits Murphy's sign, as seen in cholecystitis; place the tips of your index and middle finger at the subcostal region on the right, and ask the patient to take a deep breath in. The patient will stop breathing in as the gallbladder touches the tips of your fingers, because it causes the patient pain.
- If you are able to palpate a gallbladder, this is always pathological. If there is no coexisting jaundice, then this has resulted from obstruction of the cystic duct, resulting in a mucocoele or empyema.
- If there is co-existing jaundice, then this has resulted from obstruction of the CBD and is thought to occur due to other causes besides gallstones. With gallstones, the gallbladder wall can become thickened and fibrosed after recurrent episodes of inflammation; but gallbladder enlargement typically arises as a result of carcinoma of the head of the pancreas, or another cause as stated in Courvoisier's law.

Q3 What are the causes of abdominal ascites?
- This occurs as a result of overproduction or lack of absorption of abdominal fluid and is due to heart failure and chronic liver disease.

(Average Response)

- The causes of ascites can be divided into those that cause an exudate or a transudate:
  - **Exudate (greater than 30 g/L of protein).**
    - Peritoneal malignancy.
    - Infection, e.g. TB.
    - Obstruction of the inferior vena cava.
    - Obstruction of the hepatic portal vein.
    - Acute pancreatitis.

    – **Transudate (less than 30 g/L of protein).**
- ❑ Heart failure due to hydrostatic increase in venous return.
- ❑ Cirrhosis of liver as a result of increased portal hypertension.
- ❑ Hypoalbuminaemia due to nephrotic syndrome.

(Good Response)

Q4 What non-abdominal causes can cause abdominal pain in children?

(Honours Question)

- The differential diagnosis of abdominal pain in children includes otitis media, tonsillitis and meningitis.
- Some patients with new onset diabetes can present with abdominal pain, so always check the BM in young patients.
- **Never forget** the testicles as a possible cause leading to referred pain; remember testicular torsion is more common in children.

Children will often be vague about the site of any pain and point to the umbilicus in the majority of cases. A few tips are:
- Try to distract the child when performing the examination; the parents can often help with this.
- Ask the child to jump around; they will not do this if there is an acute abdomen.
- Use the child's own hands to palpate; place your hand above their hands and gently palpate around the abdomen.

Case 1: Organomegaly

Instructions: Please examine this abdominal mass, and tell me what you think it is.

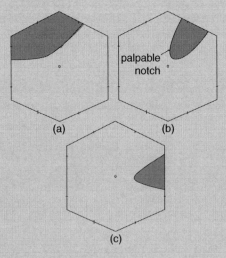

Figure 4.6a, b, c: Organomegaly

Key features to look for:

Table 4.4: Organomegaly

Variable	Liver (A)	Spleen (B)	Kidney (C)
Site	Right hypochondrium; can extend into epigastrium if very large	Left hypochondrium	Left or right flank (if very large, may involve the ipsilateral hypochondria)
Palpation	Can't get above it	Can't get above it	Can get above it
Moves with respiration	Yes	Yes, down towards RIF on inspiration	Yes, moves vertically down on inspiration
Ballotable	No	No	Yes
Percussion	Dull	Dull	Usually resonant due to overlying bowel
Special features	Can be associated with splenomegaly	Palpable notch; Enlarges towards the umbilicus/RIF	If bilateral, consider polycystic kidney disease

Completion

Organomegaly is a common examination finding in finals. You must be able to distinguish between the common abdominal viscera. If you find hepatomegaly, you must look for splenomegaly and vice versa. Other possible enlarged structures would include an AAA in the epigastrium, or a distended bladder arising from the pelvis.

Viva questions

Q1 What are the causes of hepatomegaly, splenomegaly and hepatosplenomegaly?

Table 4.5: Aetiology of organomegaly

Organomegaly	Causes
Hepatomegaly	**Jaundiced; smoothly enlarged:** Viral hepatitis, biliary tree obstruction, cholangitis **Jaundiced; knobbly enlargement:** Malignancy (primary or secondary), cirrhosis, liver abscess, hydatid cyst **No jaundice; smoothly enlarged:** Congestive cardiac failure, cirrhosis, Budd-Chiari syndrome, amyloidosis **No jaundice; knobbly enlargement:** Primary hepatocellular carcinoma, cirrhosis
Splenomegaly	**Infection:** Malaria, EBV, CMV, TB **Congestion:** Portal hypertension, congestive cardiac failure **Infarction:** Subacute bacterial endocarditis **Malignancy:** Leukaemia, lymphoma, myeloproliferative disorders **Others:** Felty's syndrome
Hepatospleno-megaly	**Infection:** Infectious mononucleosis **Cellular proliferation:** Polycythaemia rubra vera, myelofibrosis **Malignancy:** Lymphoma, leukaemia **Others:** Amyloidosis, sarcoidosis, cirrhosis

Please note this is not an exhaustive list, as there are many other causes.

Q2 What is portal hypertension?

(Difficult Question)

- This is increased portal venous pressures to >10 mm Hg.
- The most common cause worldwide is post viral hepatitis, and in the United Kingdom it is alcoholic liver cirrhosis.

Q3 What are the causes of a right iliac fossa mass?

(Difficult Question)

Table 4.6: RIF mass

Originating structure	Causes
Skin and subcutaneous tissues, muscle	Lipoma, sebaceous cyst, psoas abscess, psoas bursa
Bowel	Caecal carcinoma, Crohn's mass, TB mass, appendix abscess or mass
Urological	Transplanted kidney (most common in exam), ectopic kidney, bladder carcinoma
Reproductive system	**Males:** Ectopic testes, undescended testes **Female:** Fibroids, ovarian tumours
Blood vessels	Iliac artery aneurysms, lymphadenopathy, saphena varix, ruptured epigastric artery, femoral aneurysm

In the left iliac fossa, the causes are similar but bear in mind the possibility of a diverticular abscess or carcinoma of the colon.

4.2 DIGITAL RECTAL EXAMINATION

The rectum is approximately 12 cm in length and constitutes the terminal part of the large bowel. The rectum can be divided into thirds.

- The upper two-thirds of the rectum is covered in peritoneum; in men this peritoneum is in contact with the surface of the base of the bladder, whilst in women this peritoneum comprises the pouch of Douglas (the recto-uterine pouch) and can contain loops of bowel.
- The structures just above the first third of the rectum include:
  - **Men:** Working proximally lie the urethra, prostate, base of the bladder and seminal vesicles.
  - **Women:** The vagina and cervix (the very experienced may be able to palpate a retroverted uterus).

The rectum is continued as the anus, which is 3–4 cms in length and joins the perineum. The anus has two sets of sphincter muscles: external (voluntary) and internal (involuntary).

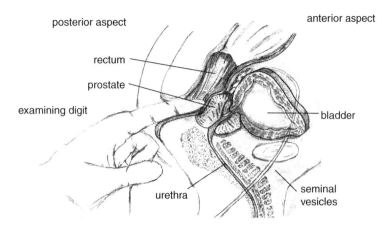

posterior aspect

anterior aspect

rectum

prostate

examining digit

bladder

urethra

seminal vesicles

Fig 4.7: The rectum

Examination of the rectum can be very revealing and is an integral part of any abdominal examination. As a junior doctor, this task is usually delegated to you, so it is important you have a good grasp of its examination. Increasingly the rectum is being examined as a separate OSCE station in its own right. You will often be asked to examine a mannequin, with the most common finding being a smoothly enlarged prostate on a male. Therefore, spend some time in your clinical skills lab, as the pathological specimens will be very similar to the ones used in the actual examination. For variation, the station may have an actor for you to interact with, but the principles of examining any system are the same.

Clinical examination

Introduction
As for any clinical encounter (*see* Chapter 1, Principles of a clinical encounter). Specifically for this case:
✔ **Explain purpose, gain consent and ask for a chaperone**
✔ **Build rapport:** It is important to get the patient to relax as much as possible, because if they don't it will make it very difficult for you to perform the examination.

Preparation
✔ **Collect your equipment**
   ■ You will need to collect disposable gloves, lubricant and some wipes.
   ■ If indicated, you must also use a stool sample tube and a faecal occult blood (FOB) strip.
✔ **Position patient appropriately**
   ■ First, **ensure privacy** by drawing a curtain around you.
   ■ Ask the patient to lie on the left-hand side facing away from you, i.e. the left lateral position, with his or her hips and knees flexed up to the chest wall and the buttocks at the edge of the examining couch.

Inspection
✔ **Inspect the perineum and anal margin**
  ▪ Part the cheeks with the fingers of one hand and inspect the perineum and anal margin, commenting on the presence of:
    – Skin tags, pilonidal sinus.
    – Anal fissures (these cause immense pain on initiation of DRE, so a suppository containing local anaesthetic should be used before conducting the examination)
    – Anal fistulae.
    – External haemorrhoids, external thrombosed piles, rectal prolapse.
    – Skin discolouration, eczema.

Palpation
✔ **Examine the anal canal**
  ▪ Warn the patient that you are about to start the intrusive part of the examination.
  ▪ Lubricate the index finger of the other hand, and press it against the posterior anal margin (at the six o'clock position).
  ▪ Then slip the lubricated finger into the anal canal, following the curve of the coccyx and sacrum upwards and backwards; feel for any obvious masses (if found, describe as you would any lump).
✔ **Examine the anterior rectal wall**
  ▪ Rotate your finger 180° by pronating at the wrist and noting the consistency of the rectal wall as you rotate your finger, you are now at the 12 o'clock position; complete the examination of the rectum by examining the entire circumference, all 360°.
  ▪ Anteriorly will be the prostate in the male, or the cervix and a retroverted uterus if present in the female. Whilst examining, note the presence of:
    – **Lumps/masses:** A carcinoma will be palpable as an irregular mass; there may be faeces present in constipation, which will be indentable on examination.
    – **Tenderness:** This may be present in cases of pelvic appendicitis; in women, comment on whether you can elicit any tenderness whilst palpating the cervix anteriorly; this may indicate the presence of endometriosis in the pouch of Douglas.
    – **Haemorrhoids:** Only palpable when thrombosed.
    – **Ballooning of the rectal cavity:** Present in proximal obstructions to the rectum.
✔ **Examine the prostate**

Remember that the normal prostate measures approximately 3.5 cm in width and will protrude approximately 1 cm into the lumen. The normal consistency is rubbery with a smooth surface and a palpable sulcus between the two lobes.
  ▪ **Surface:** Is the surface irregular, craggy, hard, or are there any palpable lumps? All suggest carcinoma of the prostate gland.
  ▪ **Size:** Is the gland generally enlarged? Can you feel a palpable sulcus? Obliteration suggests gross enlargement, secondary to a malignancy. If the enlargement is symmetrical, this suggests prostatic hypertrophy.
  ▪ **Tenderness:** If there is any tenderness on palpation of the prostate, this suggests prostatitis.

✔ **Assess for anal tone**
- You can ask the patient to bear down on your finger now to assess the anaₗ if appropriate.
- This is useful in cases of faecal incontinence or neurological disease. This proceᵤᵤₑ also helps assess any lesions in the upper rectum missed by the examining finger, which moves caudally.

✔ **Inspect the examining finger**
- Remove your finger; note the presence of faeces, blood or mucus on the examining finger.

Complete the examination

✔ **Thank the patient**
- Wipe the examining surface of the patient, cover him or her with a sheet and leave the patient in privacy to dress.

✔ **Wash your hands**

✔ **Complete further examination**
- *'To complete my examination, I would like to examine the abdomen and send off a stool sample for faecal occult blood'.*

A stool sample for FOB testing is often sent in combination with the DRE to help with the diagnosis of anaemia or GI bleeding.

✔ **Present your findings**

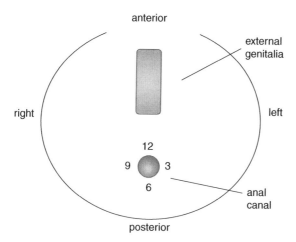

Figure 4.8: Lithotomy position

- Turn to the examiner and present your examination findings, which are described in relation to an imaginary clock face in the lithotomy position, i.e. 12 o'clock is anterior, and six o'clock is posterior.
- Begin with what you noted on external inspection first, followed by internal examination.

There is usually never a good reason not to examine the rectum as a surgeon. Apart from patient refusal, the only situations where it may be excusable are in children, as it adds very little to your clinical assessment, and in adults where examination causes undue pain and you are unable to continue. In the latter case, an examination under anaesthesia needs to be considered.

Viva questions

Q1 What are the indications for performing a DRE?
- **Acute abdomen assessment:** Appendicitis, peritonitis, lower abdominal pain.
- **Prostate assessment:** In patients with symptoms of prostatic hypertrophy or suspicion of prostatic carcinoma.
- **Pre-procedure:** Prior to invasive procedures assessing the bowel including proctoscopy, sigmoidoscopy and colonoscopy.
- **Diagnostic purposes:**
  - **Constipation:** To assess for presence of faeces in the rectum.
  - **Change in bowel habit:** There may be a palpable anal or rectal tumour.
  - Anorectal pain or tenesmus.
  - In cases of iron deficiency anaemia to exclude malignancy or bleeding.
  - Symptoms related to urinary/faecal continence.

Q2 What are haemorrhoids?
These are enlarged anal cushions.

(Surgical Definition)

Patients typically present with a history of painless, bright red rectal bleeding; however, haemorrhoids can be painful if they have thrombosed.

Q3 How are haemorrhoids managed?

(Difficult Question)

- **Conservatively:**
  - Sitz baths, analgesia and dietary advice.
  - **Injection sclerotherapy:** A Gabriel syringe containing 5% phenol in almond oil is injected into the haemorrhoid above the dentate line. In men it is important to be aware of inadvertent injection into the prostate gland, causing prostatitis.
  - **Banding:** A rubber band is placed around the pile, which causes ischaemia and shrinkage.
- **Surgical:** Haemorrhoidectomy.

The dentate line is an anatomical landmark that divides the sensory part of the anal canal. Above it there is no sensation, but below it there *is* sensation, and therefore the patient will feel pain if you try to inject haemorrhoids below this line.

4.3 ABDOMINAL STOMA EXAMINATION

The examination of a stoma, if present, can be very revealing about a patient's operative management. You may simply be asked to comment on the stoma or be asked to
specifically examine it. Most students often say they have no idea how to examine a
stoma, when in fact they could probably describe the majority of the features that are
examined for. The key is to demonstrate this in a logical manner and to be confident in
your approach. The majority of your examination focuses on inspection alone, so just
say what you see.

Authors' Top Tip

*We advise you to spend an afternoon with the stoma care nurse on her rounds, as you will see
a competent stoma examination and see the many different types of stomas available.*

Do not remove the stoma bag in the examination unless you have been specifically
directed to do so.

Clinical examination

Introduction
As for any clinical encounter (*see* Chapter 1, Principles of a clinical encounter).

Inspection
✔ **Describe the site of the stoma**
  ▪ This is the most crucial part of the examination, as often the site will tell you what
    the stoma type is; a stoma in the left iliac fossa is typically a colostomy, whereas
    an ileostomy is found in the RIF.

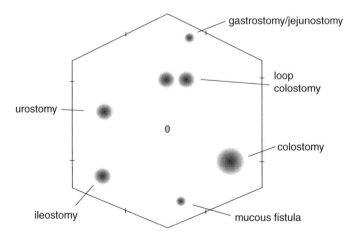

Figure 4.9: Sites of common stomas

✔ **Estimate the size of the lumen**
  ■ The size of the lumen will help determine the type:
    – **Large calibre:** Colostomy.
    – **Small calibre:** Ileostomy or urostomy.
  ■ If the lumen is small, this may have occurred from complications related to stomas, such as stenosis or retraction. A prolapsed stoma will make the lumen look bigger.
✔ **Count the number of lumens**
  ■ **Single lumen:** In most cases it is a single lumen, i.e. an end stoma.
  ■ **Double lumen:** This may be a looped or double stoma.

Do not be caught out by the situation where there is more than one stoma, e.g. a colostomy and a mucous fistula.

✔ **Examine for a spout**
  ■ **Absence of spout:** If the lumen is flush with the skin, it is probably a colostomy (unless prolapsed).
  ■ **Spout present:** Ileostomies have a spout to keep the irritant effluent off the skin. Urostomies also have a spout.
✔ **Examine bag effluent**
  ■ Look at the contents for the following:

Bag content:
    – **Dark-green fluid:** Ileostomy.
    – **Solid faeces:** Colostomy.
    – **Urine:** Urostomy.

Odour: Faeculent in colostomies, and odourless in ileostomies.

✔ **Look for abdominal scars**
  ■ The scars may give you a clue as to what surgery the patient had, e.g. usually you will see a midline laparotomy scar in conjunction with a colostomy, which can be from an abdominoperineal resection or a Hartmann's procedure.
  ■ There may be evidence of surgical closure of previous stomas.

Complete the examination
✔ **Thank the patient**
✔ **Wash your hands**
✔ **Further examination**
  ■ *'To complete my examination, I would like to examine the perineum to look for the presence of a patent anal canal and anal stump. I would also like to examine for complications of the stoma'.*

In the case of a colostomy stoma, the presence of a patent anal canal or closed perineum will help you differentiate between an abdominoperineal resection and a Hartmann's procedure on clinical examination. If the perineum is closed, then it is an abdomino-perineal resection, which is usually performed for a low-lying rectal cancer or severe ulcerative colitis. Usually it is sufficient to tell the examiner that you would ask the patient if he or she has an anal canal, which if present suggests the patient had a Hartmann's procedure. This would usually have been done as an emergency for diverticulitis or bowel obstruction, secondary to a colorectal cancer.

✔ Present your findings

Viva questions

Q1 What is a stoma?
This is a surgically created connection between the GI tract and the skin. It can be temporary (reversible) or permanent.

(Surgical Definition)

Q2 How would you distinguish between an ileostomy and colostomy?

(Difficult Question)

Table 4.7: Ileostomy and colostomy

Clinical Feature	Ileostomy	Colostomy
Site	RIF	LIF
Presence of spout	Spouted	Flush
Bag effluent	Odourless, dark-green liquid	Solid faeces
Effluent volume	500 mL (low output) to 1 L (high output) per day	300 mL/day

Q3 What are the complications of a stoma?

(Difficult Question)

This can be divided into general complications and complications specific to the stoma itself:

- **General complications:** Nutritional disorders, e.g. vitamin B deficiency, renal stones, short gut syndrome, stoma diarrhoea, psychological.
- **Specific complications:** Technical problems such as ischaemia, prolapse, parastomal hernia, stenosis or retraction. Practical problems include malodour, skin irritation due to spillage of bag effluent.

Q4 What are the causes of abdominal pain?

Abdominal pain is frequently encountered in both primary and secondary care settings and is often challenging to the physician, representing the top three presentations to the emergency department. In the majority of cases the pain is related to benign aetiology; however, in some cases it can be related to more serious conditions.

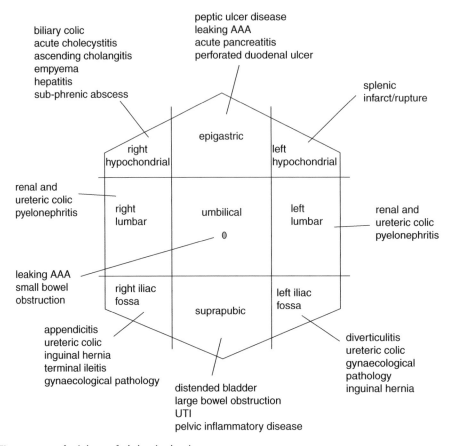

Figure 4.10: Aetiology of abdominal pain

Pain can be categorised depending on its aetiology:

- **Visceral pain:** Diffuse pain that is poorly localised; usually described as being dull and aching in character.
  - Foregut pain is described as being epigastric in site.
  - Mid-gut pain is usually felt in the para-umbilical region.
  - Hindgut pain is described as pain in the lower abdomen.
- **Parietal/somatic pain:** Well-localised and sharp in nature, arising from peritoneal inflammation.
- **Referred pain:** Aching in nature and perceived as being near the surface of the body.

Q5   What are the indications for the various types of stoma?

(Honours Question)

Table 4.8: Stoma indications

Indication	Examples
Feeding	Jejunostomy, gastrostomy.
Decompression	Caecostomy, gastrostomy.
Diversion	**Urostomy (Ileal Conduit):** After cystectomy, a loop of ileum may be used for urinary diversion, in which the ureters are anastomosed to one end of the loop, with the other end brought out as a urostomy. **Ileostomy:** This could be a temporary manoeuvre in order to protect a distal anastomosis, allowing it time to heal; or it could be permanent in cases of IBD, in which it rests the bowel. **Loop colostomy:** These are currently performed using the sigmoid colon. Once the bowel is brought to the surface, the wall is partially cut to produce two separate openings, one which functions to allow the release of stool and gas, and the other which is non-functioning. **Double-barrelled colostomy:** Both ends of the colon are brought to the surface next to each other and are sutured together along the anti-mesenteric border.
Exteriorisation	**Double-barrelled colostomy: See above.** **End Colostomy:** This can also be either temporary or permanent; permanent being most often after an abdominoperineal resection. **End colostomy and rectal stump:** Known as a Hartmann's procedure, the proximal end of the large bowel is brought to the surface (usually in the LIF) and the rectal stump is oversewn. Normally done for tumours of the rectum or anus. **End colostomy and mucous fistula:** In this uncommon procedure, both ends of the bowel are brought to the surface separately as stomas; however, the distal end is small and non-functioning, only producing mucous, and the proximal end of the bowel allows the passage of stool and gas. This procedure makes it easier to access the distal end of the bowel and therefore sew the two ends back together in the future.

CHAPTER 5

Lumps and bumps: breast lumps

5.1 LUMPS AND BUMPS

This forms the majority of short cases you are likely to see in finals. Increasingly, it is becoming an OSCE station in its own right.

Authors' Top Tip

Sometimes the diagnosis is obvious and you may offer a spot diagnosis. However, be wary of this, and unless otherwise directed avoid this approach as you may lose out on easy points; remember that the examiners can only mark you on what you say or do.

We will begin by explaining how you would describe any common lump, then follow with features of the common lumps and bumps that you are likely to encounter on the body. For specific regional lumps such as those found on the neck or breast, the principles are the same; be systematic and you will score the relevant points.

Clinical examination

Introduction

As for any clinical encounter (*see* Chapter 1, Principles of a clinical encounter).

Inspection
✔ **Describe observable features**
  - **Site:** This will give you a clue to the diagnosis, e.g. a sebaceous cyst in hair-bearing areas. For lumps in body areas that are not commonly amenable to regional descriptive terms, it is acceptable to measure a distance from a fixed anatomical landmark and describe the lump site with respect to this, e.g. *the lump is 5 cm proximal to…or on the dorsal aspect of…*
  - **Size:** Two-dimensional estimates in centimetres are a minimum, although technically a lump is a three-dimensional lesion.
  - **Number:** Remember, there may be more than one lump, and in the case of lymph nodes, several. Don't bother counting all the lumps, simply say: 'There are multiple lumps'.

- **Shape:** Is it spherical, oval, etc.?
- **Colour:** Overlying erythema or abnormal skin colour.
- **Transillumination:** With a pen torch, see if the mass is fluid or solid.

Authors' Top Tip

Traditionally it has been taught that to truly transilluminate a lump, you must place a light source on one side of the lump and an opaque tube on the other side; if transilluminable, the light source should shine through to the opaque tube. We have seen candidates use a variety of opaque tubes for this purpose, the most popular being the Smarties tube. We suggest you avoid this for several reasons. Firstly, if a lump is truly transilluminable and the examiner wishes you to demonstrate this, in the examination this will usually be obvious and simply shining a torch onto the lump will cause it to glow even without the opaque tube. Secondly, in some situations it is best to use you own hand as the opaque tube, this is especially true with scrotal swellings. And so we advise you stay clear of any tricks anyone has taught you to demonstrate transilluminability. Keep it simple.

Palpation

✔ **Check for tenderness**
  - Whether a lump is painful or not is a useful clue, e.g. the painful benign breast lump versus the painless malignant lump.

✔ **Check the temperature**
  - The temperature of the overlying skin may be warm in acute inflammatory lesions or vascular lesions.

✔ **Examine the edge**
  - Are there well-defined, clear margins, or is the lump diffuse with no discernable edge?

✔ **Examine the consistency**
  - Is the lump hard, rubbery or soft?
  - Is the surface smooth or nodular?

✔ **Check for fluctuance**
  - Place two fingers on either side of the lump. With your other hand, press down in the middle of the lump, perpendicular to your resting fingers, and squash the lump.
  - If your resting fingers move apart as a result, this suggests the lump is fluctuant, although this must be repeated to confirm – this time with the resting fingers surrounding the lump at right angles to their initial position.
  - If the lump is fluctuant, this suggests the lump is fluid-filled; lipomas are often fluctuant due to their fat content.

✔ **Check for compressibility**
  - With the flat of your middle three fingers, gently squash the lump and hold.
  - If the lump disappears completely but then reappears immediately after you let go, then the lump is said to be compressible.
  - This is often seen in vascular structures, such as AV malformations or a saphena varix, as the structures' fluid content empties with compression but refills when the pressure is released.

Authors' Top Tip

Students often misunderstand the terms fluctuance and compressibility. If you follow the above descriptions, you should not make this common mistake. However, we suggest you get your surgical tutors to demonstrate this to you, as the concept may be difficult to grasp initially.

✔ **Check for pulsatility**
  ▪ Remember, a lump may be pulsatile simply because it lies over an artery and is therefore termed as having a transmitted pulsatility. To demonstrate pulsatility, place two fingers over the lump, which will move up and down with each pulsation.
  ▪ You may also need to check if the lump is pulsatile and expansile, as this can indicate an aneurysm or vascular malformation. To demonstrate expansibility, place one finger on either side of the lump, and you will see your fingers moving laterally with each pulse.
✔ **Assess fixity (or mobility)**
  ▪ You can check specifically to see if a lump is attached to a specific anatomical plane, be it skin or the underlying muscle; this helps identify the lesion and can suggest malignancy.
  ▪ **Skin:** This will help determine the lump's origin:
    – With the flat of your fingers, try and move the skin over the lump. If the overlying skin is freely mobile, then the lump is separate from the skin and therefore originates deep to the skin. If the skin puckers instead, this is called tethering.
    – Now move the lump itself and see how the overlying skin moves with it. If the lump moves with the skin, this suggests the lump originates from the skin, e.g. a sebaceous cyst.
  ▪ **Muscle:** This requires an appreciation of the direction of the underlying muscle fibres, as you will need to move the lump parallel and perpendicular to these underlying fibres.
    – First, grasp the lump between your thumb and index finger, then move the lump in two perpendicular planes. Is this freely mobile?
    – Repeat the manoeuvre, but this time ask the patient to tense the underlying muscle (the method for this depends on the underlying muscle group you are examining). Is the lump now fixed? Fixity to this suggests invasion of the lump into the muscle and that the lump is likely to be malignant rather than benign. If the lump is freely mobile, then the lump is considered to be superficial to the muscle.

We prefer to use the term fixity rather than mobility, as really what you are looking for is not if a lump is mobile. Although this can be useful in the case of a very mobile breast lump suggesting a fibroadenoma, you are more concerned with whether a lump is fixed to any underlying anatomical structure, be it skin or muscle, as this is highly suggestive of malignant disease.

Auscultation

✔ **Auscultate for a bruit**
- The site of the lump will help you decide if this is necessary, and often other features will help you decide if you think the structure may be vascular, such as pulsatility in the neck.
- The AV renal dialysis fistula at the wrist is usually an obvious spot diagnosis; in this case you would listen for a machinery murmur.

Percussion adds very little to your examination unless you believe the lump may be an organ, whether bowel or renal transplant. For these situations, follow the specific regional examination schema instead of the generic one outlined above.

Complete the examination

✔ **Further examination**
- *'To complete my examination I would like to examine the distal neurology, vascular supply and the regional lymphatic chain'.*
- The lymphatic chain you examine would depend on the site of the lump, e.g. in the case of a neck lump, the local lymph nodes would be the cervical lymphatic chains. If the lump you were examining is an enlarged lymph node you would be expected to say that you would also examine the lymphoreticular system, i.e. check for generalised lymphadenopathy and hepatosplenomegaly.
✔ **Thank the patient**
✔ **Wash your hands**
✔ **Present your findings**

There are some specific features in examining a lump that are only relevant according to the specific case; therefore we have not discussed these above. These ommissions include reducibility, percussion for resonance or palpation for a cough impulse, which are commonly used in the examination of a groin lump, as these may suggest a hernia. For such

Table 5.1: Common lumps

Features	Lipoma	Sebaceous cyst	Lymph node
Site	Any region where there is fat	Hair-bearing areas	Lymphatic chains
Consistency	Soft	Hard/firm	Hard/firm/rubbery
Edge	Ill-defined edges; slip sign (lump tends to move away from examining finger)	Well-demarcated	Usually well-demarcated unless matted together, in which case it would be indistinct
Fluctuant	Yes	No	No
Fixity	Mobile freely; overlying skin freely mobile	Lump moves with skin; overlying skin not freely mobile	Lump fixed deeply; overlying skin mobile; tethering in TB or malignancy; lymphoma may be mobile
Special features	If you have found one, look for others: multiple lipomas suggest Dercum's disease	Visible punctum with toothpaste-like discharge (sebum)	May be multiple, matted together; overlying skin changes, e.g. erythema in TB

specific regional lump cases, we advise you follow the various schema suggested in the following few chapters with the above principles in mind.

Remember, these lumps can appear anywhere and range from a lump in the neck to a lump in the groin. So, bear this is mind whenever you examine a lump on the body or trunk. Always ask yourself if it could be a lymph node, a lipoma or a sebaceous cyst before you consider an alternative diagnosis.

Examiner's Anecdote

'He gave me an absolutely classic description of a sebaceous cyst when he examined the woman's breast but decided to ignore his findings and instead discussed breast cancer management. Never forget that common lumps such as lipomas or sebaceous cysts can also occur on the breast, so always consider these in your differentials'.

The main point to consider when differentiating between a lipoma and a sebaceous cyst is its location in hair-bearing areas, its toothpaste-like discharge and the presence of a visible punctum (50%), which if found is virtually pathognomonic of a sebaceous cyst.

Many students surprisingly ask what we mean by hair-bearing areas. Aside from the obvious sites of the scalp, neck, shoulders, back and groin, including the scrotum, generally this means areas of the body where sebaceous cysts are likely to occur, i.e. wherever there are sebaceous glands. This therefore excludes the palms of the hand and soles of the feet.

If your diagnosis is lymphadenopathy, you must offer to examine the lymphoreticular system. This will include checking for hepatosplenomegaly and lymphadenopathy elsewhere, particularly the axillary and groin regions, in addition to checking the patient's FBC and LDH levels and requesting a CXR to exclude a possible lymphoma.

Viva questions

Q1 This woman has a lump in the popliteal fossa; what is it?

(Difficult Question)

This question was asked in one of the author's finals examination. It is easy to be flustered by this kind of question, especially in a stressful situation. Do not let yourself down and do not be bullied into banking on a single diagnosis. For those of you who would have said Baker's cyst without thinking about it, your answer would've been considered an average response; although in this particular case it was the wrong answer. Be systematic and logical; this question is what we call gold dust. This is because although on the surface it seems like an orthopaedic question, the principles behind the answer may well be used to differentiate between the average student and the top students. The answer is actually very easy, so long as you are logical.

The examiner will be impressed that you have started an intelligent discussion without just answering his question outright. Even if you have no idea what the answer is, you would be well on your way to scoring the majority of your marks simply by following this well-known surgical sieve. For the cause of a lump in any region, we have advised and will continue to advise particularly if you are unsure of the diagnosis to consider the differentials in terms of the structures found in that region, from superficial to deep.

- **Skin and subcutaneous tissues:** Sebaceous cyst or lipoma.
- **Vascular:** DVT, saphena varix of the SPJ junction; popliteal artery aneurysm.
- **Nerve:** Tibial nerve neuroma.
- **Bursa:** Enlarged, semi-membranous bursa.
- **Synovial fluid structures:** Baker's or popliteal cyst.

If you are still unsure, send the patient for a USS, which can accurately identify a Baker's cyst.

Q2 What is a cyst?

A cyst is a fluid-filled cavity lined by epithelium (or endothelium).

(Surgical Definition)

Case 1: Ganglion

Instructions: Please examine this lump and inform me of your diagnosis.

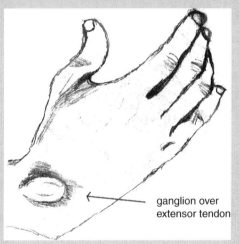

ganglion over
extensor tendon

Figure 5.1: Ganglion

Key features to look for:

Inspection
- **Site:** Lump associated with a tendon or joint (synovial-lined cavity); in this case the wrist joint on the extensor aspect.
- **Edge:** Well-defined.

Palpation
- **Consistency:** Firm/tense but may be soft if very large; as it contains fluid, it can be fluctuant, especially if large.
- **Fixity:** Lump moves with the tendon; in this case, if you flex the wrist it makes the lump more prominent; overlying skin freely mobile.

Completion

'There is a 2-cm, well-defined, tense swelling over the extensor aspect of the wrist. It appears to move along the line of the extensor tendon with the overlying skin also freely mobile. The most likely diagnosis is that of a ganglion'.

Ganglia are commonly found around the wrists and ankle but can be found almost anywhere in the body, although they are typically associated with anatomical structures that are lined with synovium. The above case is essentially a spot diagnosis, but you should still try and describe the lump as fully as possible; remember you may be referring this patient to a surgeon on the phone, and he cannot spot your diagnosis as being clearly correct.

Viva questions

Q1   What is a ganglion?

This is a cystic degeneration of the tendon sheath (or joint capsule). It leads to a communication with the synovium, which contains gelatinous fluid.

(Surgical Definition)

Q2   How would you treat this?

Through conservative measures and surgical measures:

Conservative

- ■ Aspiration and immobilisation; however, there is a risk of recurrence.
- ■ Nothing (in asymptomatic patients).

Surgical

- ■ Excision.

Authors' Top Tip

You may have heard of the 'Bible striking the ganglion to cure it'; we advise you not to mention this to the examiner.

5.2   BREAST

The breast is made up of glandular tissue, fibrous connective tissue, fatty tissue, nerves, blood vessels and lymph nodes.

Breast lumps are common; the majority (90%) are benign. Many patients present after having felt or noticed changes in the breast; the remaining are referred from screening services. Breast cancer is the commonest malignancy in the female population and hence of great clinical importance. The lifetime risk of developing breast cancer is one in 10, and the risk rises significantly from 30 to 50 years of age. Breast cancer does occur in men, but it is rare, and where suspected urgent referral is indicated. Breast cancer is easier to treat the earlier it is identified, as there are more treatment options available.

Despite its obvious limitations, breast examination is something no student should be unable to perform confidently; you are bound to have a case in finals. There is an abundance of imitation breast models in medical schools to practise with. Often, these contain the sorts of lumps you will see during finals, and sometimes the same equipment is even used in the actual OSCE. However, do not lull yourself into a false sense of security; increasingly in medical school exams you may find, as one of the author's did (much to his surprise!), an actual female breast to examine, which coincidentally did have a lump!

Clinical examination

Introduction

As for any clinical encounter, (*see* Chapter 1, Principles of a clinical encounter). Specifically for this case:

- **Explain purpose, gain consent and ask for a chaperone**.
- **Build rapport:** Inform patient of what you are doing as you go along; remember, you are going to be examining the patient's breast. This is an intimate and intrusive examination that may be uncomfortable, so be gentle and ask about pain as necessary.

Medicolegally, you are obliged to offer a chaperone, even if you are female. It is not only good clinical practise but is in accordance with GMC guidelines. If the patient refuses a chaperone, which they are entitled to, then you must clearly document this in your notes. Do not accept family members as chaperones; always have a third-party present, often a female nurse, and document her full name, position and the patient's consent for the party to be present.

Authors' Top Tip

Increasingly, medical schools are now incorporating the request for a chaperone in the examination into the actual mark scheme. So it is not enough to say that you would offer the patient a chaperone, you must physically turn to the examiner and specifically ask for one. The examiner will almost certainly say that he or she will act as your chaperone.

Inspection

It is perfectly acceptable to ask the patient if she has noticed any lumps or nipple discharge. This is because you would not be expected to express nipple discharge in the OSCE, as this can be uncomfortable for the patient. In the clinical setting, it is kinder to ask them to express this and take note of the colour and whether it is coming from a single duct or multiple ducts.

We find it is easier to ask about this when you enquire about pain in the breasts before palpation. This also helps you focus your examination to the side of pathology after having examined the normal side.

5.2.1 General inspection

With the patient sitting on the edge of the bed and her hands relaxed by her side, look for and comment on the following features:

- **Scars:** Mastectomy from previous breast carcinoma with associated arm lymphoedema caused by axillary node clearance; say you would check the abdomen and back for a scar if there was evidence of breast reconstruction (*see* Viva Q8); also look underneath the breast for scars from breast implant surgery.
- **Lumps:** Any obvious lumps (unlikely); describe as for any lump on inspection.
- **Asymmetry:** Size or contour of the breast; often breasts are normally slightly asymmetrical in size.
- **Skin changes:** Dimpling caused by infiltration of the dermis by the tumour, peau d'orange suggesting presence of an aggressive tumour, puckering, erythema, oedema caused by blockage of the intramammary lymphatics, ulceration from cancer; radiotherapy ink marks from previous treatment.
- **Nipple signs:** Retraction or inversion caused by periductal inflammation and fibrosis, and whether it is unilateral, as seen in carcinoma, or bilateral, which is characteristic of benign nipple inversion; nipple eczema, especially unilateral, suggests Paget's disease; if bilateral it may be part of a generalised skin condition. Also, note the presence of any nipple discharge.
- **General features:** Cachexia or lymphoedema of the upper arm suggests either metastatic spread or axillary lymph node clearance following a woman's previous mastectomy for breast malignancy.

If the woman has large, pendulous breasts, then it is acceptable to lift the breast (with permission) to look underneath for any abnormalities such as eczema, cellulitis or scars.

✔ Special manoeuvres
Inspect for any previously missed abnormalities:
- **Hands on hips:** With the patient's hands pushed in to the side of the hips, thereby contracting the pectoralis major muscle, this makes skin dimpling or tethering more obvious.
- **Arm raise:** With the patient's arms raised above her head, this strains the ligaments of Astley Cooper and stretches the pectoral muscles, allowing a better view of the inframammary area. It also accentuates asymmetry and skin tethering.

Palpation
Palpation is done with the patient in a supine position, the head supported with a pillow and both arms raised above the head to distribute the breast tissue more evenly for palpation. Ensure you examine both breasts and start with the normal side.

✔ Palpate the breasts

There are many techniques for palpation, ranging from concentric circles beginning at the nipple and moving outwards or by systematically examining with the flat of your fingers in four imaginary quadrants. Although equally acceptable, we typically use both methods. Whichever method you use, bear in mind the commonly described breast quadrants.

The breast is split into several regions: areola, nipple, axillary tail and the four regional quadrants. The upper outer quadrant is the most common site of malignancy.

Your field of palpation will involve the region between the clavicle superiorly and the inframammary fold inferiorly, your medial landmark will be the sternum and your

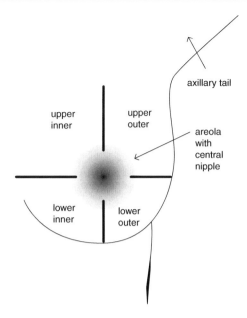

Figure 5.2: Breast quadrants

field of palpation will extend laterally to the mid-axillary line including the tail of breast tissue extending into the axilla.

Be systematic in your examination, so as not to miss anything. Palpation is normally done with the flat of the index, middle and ring fingers held together, covering small sections at a time. First, palpate lightly and then repeat palpation over the same region, pressing more deeply. We suggest the following sequence:

- **Field of palpation.**
  - **Nipple and areola:** Note that candidates often forget this region.
  - Breast quadrants.
  - Axillary tail.
- **Palpation techniques.**
  - Palpating in concentric circles, starting at the nipple and working in concentric circles to the periphery.
  - Palpating in overlapping vertical strips across the entire field.
  - Starting at the periphery, palpate section by section to the nipple in a radial fashion, repeating until all four quadrants of the breast are palpated.

✔ **Assess the breast lump**

If you find a lump, consider the following:

- **Describe the lump:** Do this as you would any lump, e.g. site, size, etc.
- **Assess fixity:**
  - Whilst you are holding the lump between the pulps of your index finger and thumb, see if you can move the lump at right angles and parallel to the muscle fibres; if you can't do this, then the lump is fixed (suggesting malignancy). If you can move the lump, then it is mobile (usually benign).

－ Now, ask the patient to place her hands on her hips and push in, tensing her chest muscles. Repeat the manoeuvre, checking for fixity with the underlying pectoralis major muscle.

Authors' Top Tip

Another popular method for assessing fixity is to ask the patient to push against your resisting hand with her ipsilateral arm.

✔ **Check for regional lymphadenopathy**
  ■ **Cervical region.**
  ■ **Supraclavicular region.**
  ■ **Axillary region.**
    － This can either be done with the patient either lying down or sitting up.
    － Support the patient's right arm with *your* right arm to relax her muscles, and with the left hand palpate systematically starting in the apex of the axilla and working your way around the four axillary walls (anterior, posterior, medial chest walls and laterally).
    － The presence of nodes in any of these regions may suggest metastatic disease.
    － Describe the nodes in terms of their site (apical, medial, lateral, anterior or posterior nodal groups in the axillary chain), the number of nodes palpable, their consistency and mobility.

Complete the examination
✔ **Further examination**
  ■ *'To complete my examination, I would like to auscultate the chest for an effusion, examine the abdomen for hepatomegaly and assess the spine for percussion tenderness'.*

If you suspect malignancy, you must examine the chest, liver and bony spine, as these are the most common sites for breast metastases.

✔ **Thank the patient:** Ensure the patient is comfortable, and ask her to redress or offer a blanket to cover up.
✔ **Wash your hands**
✔ **Present your findings, e.g.:**

'On examination, there is a 1 cm by 1 cm, well-defined, mobile lump in the inner outer quadrant of the right breast, which is soft, smooth and non-tender. There is no underlying chest wall fixation and no palpable axillary, cervical or supraclavicular lymphadenopathy. Systemic examination reveals no evidence of malignant spread. The most likely diagnosis is that of a benign breast lump, such as a fibroadenoma, but my differential diagnosis would include a cyst. As with any breast lump, I would like to exclude a breast carcinoma, therefore I would like to complete my triple assessment with a thorough clinical history, a mammogram (or USS breast) and a fine-needle aspiration of the lump sent off for cytology'.

> ### Authors' Top Tip
>
> *Ensure you mention triple assessment at some point in your OSCE, as this key term is likely to score you extra points with the examiner.*

The key for the examination is whether you can differentiate on clinical examination between a suspicious breast lump and a benign lump. Although almost all patients get triple assessment, this does not excuse you from having developed clinical skills to risk-prioritise patients.

Table 5.2: Benign and malignant breast lumps

Clinical features	Malignant lump	Benign lump
Tenderness	No	Yes
Discharge	Unilateral, can be bloody	Bilateral, no blood, green-yellow colour
Nipple/skin changes	Nipple retraction, skin dimpling, p'eau d'orange appearance	No
Margins	Irregular	Smooth
Consistency	Hard	Rubbery, firm
Fixation	Yes	No

You are unlikely to have or require a great deal of understanding regarding the various types of mastectomies or breast surgery options available. It is, however, important that you are aware of the commonly performed wide, local excision in breast conservation therapy and of axillary node clearance and their complications, such as lymphoedema and winging of the scapula, secondary to damage to the long thoracic nerve.

Know that sentinel node biopsy is gaining popularity. This is when the first regional draining node is sampled for disease, and if negative, obviates the need for lymph node clearance, thereby reducing the morbidity associated with the procedure.

Viva questions

Q1 What is triple assessment?
- History and clinical examination.
- Imaging with either USS or mammogram.
- Biopsy with FNA for cytology, or core biopsy for histological diagnosis and immunohistochemistry studies to determine oestrogen and progesterone receptor status of the tumour.

Q2 What image modalities will you use in this patient?

(Difficult Question)

- USS is usually done in the younger patient population (<35 years); this is because their breasts contain more glandular tissue, which tends to be more dense and so reduces mammographic sensitivity.

- Mammograms are (as part of the national screening programme) usually performed in patients >35 years of age (note: two views are taken; oblique and craniocaudal).
- If the woman has small breasts, then USS is preferred, as it is physically difficult to perform a mammogram.
- An MRI is used when USS or mammograms are unhelpful; MRIs can also be used in patients with breast implants, where USS is not particularly helpful.

Q3 What is the National Breast Screening Programme?

(Difficult Question)

- This national programme in the United Kingdom was initially the first in the world, and it is aimed at detecting breast cancer in its early stages. It is open to all women between the ages of 50–70 years for routine single oblique mammography every 3 years. It was set up by the DoH in 1988. To learn more about this, read *The Forrest Report*.
- It is hoped that by the year 2012, the age for patients being invited for screening will be extended to 47–73 years. The programme is estimated to save the lives of over 1 000 women each year in the United Kingdom.

Q4 If you were concerned about metastasis associated with breast cancer, what sort of staging tests would you request?
- **FBC:** To look for bone marrow involvement suggested by anaemia and leucopenia.
- **LFTs:** Raised ALT, Gamma-GT and calcium indicate liver and bone metastases.
- **CXR:** To look for an effusion and metastases.
- **Isotope bone scan, liver USS and CT chest/abdomen:** To look for metastases.

Q5 How would you differentiate between Paget's disease of the breast and eczema?
- Paget's disease tends be unilateral, is not itchy and has no vesicular rash.
- If the areola area is affected rather than the nipple, then this suggests eczema.

In all cases, however, the patient is sent for imaging and biopsy to confirm. Paget's disease is an intraductal carcinoma of the breast.

Q6 What is the difference between tethering and fixation?

(Difficult Question)

- A lump that is fixed is immobile, whilst a tethered lump has some mobility.
- A fixed lump has infiltrated the skin, whereas tethering infiltrates along the ligaments of Astley Cooper.
- The overlying skin of a fixed lump cannot be moved over the lump, whereas the skin will dimple at the extremes of movement in a tethered lump.
- A fixed lump has a worse prognosis than a tethered lump.

Q7 What are the borders of the axilla?

(Difficult Question)

- **Anteriorly:** Pectoralis major and minor.
- **Medially:** Serratus anterior.
- **Posteriorly:** Subscapularis and teres major.
- **Laterally:** The convergence of the anterior and posterior borders at the humeral bicipital groove.
- **The apex:** The first rib, scapula and clavicle.
- **The floor:** Skin and axillary fascia.

Q8   This woman has had breast reconstruction; can you tell which operation she has had?

(Honours Question)

Aside from implants, prostheses or tissue expanders, there are two main procedures using myocutaneous flaps:

- **Transverse rectus abdominis myocutaneous (TRAM) flap:** Ovoid-shaped breast scar and horizontal scar across the abdomen.
- **The latissimus dorsi flap:** Breast scar and scar over the back.

Nipple reconstruction is usually done later, often 6 months post-surgery, so do not be surprised if you see no nipple in the examination.

CHAPTER 6

Lumps and bumps: neck lumps and thyroid

The most common cause of a neck lump is cervical lymphadenopathy. However, in clinical exams the most likely case you will encounter is a thyroid goitre.

There are other miscellaneous lumps that could come up but are less likely. Typically, they form short cases whereby you examine the lump as you would examine any general lump (*see* Chapter 5, Lumps and bumps) bearing in mind specific features depending on the case presented. Remember, as with any region, lumps such as sebaceous cysts and lipomas can also occur, so bear these in mind whenever discussing your differential diagnosis.

6.1 NECK LUMPS

Neck lumps are common, and although in some cases they may represent a more serious disease process, most of the time they are benign. In adults older than 40 years, lateral neck lumps are thought to be cancer until proved otherwise. In children and adults up to the age of 40 years, neck lumps are usually secondary to an infective process; the next most common cause is congenital, followed by a malignant cause. You must undertake the following steps to reach a diagnosis:

1. A thorough but focused clinical history.
2. Examination of the head and neck; ENT exam.
3. FNA and possibly a CT scan.

During history-taking, it is important to ascertain the length of time the swelling has been present, and whether it has changed over that time period. If the lump has appeared acutely, increased in size and is painful, this suggests an inflammatory process as opposed to a slow-growing, painless lesion, which is more suggestive of a malignant cause. If you suspect an inflammatory process has caused the lump, examination of the ear, nose and throat (ENT) is essential to assess for infection.

The duration of time the neck lump has been present is important, as most inflammatory lumps will disappear within a few weeks, whereas a persistent lump will require referral to an ENT surgeon.

Authors' Top Tip

A golden rule to remember for your careers as junior doctors: *Any neck lump you are considering excising should be formally assessed by an ENT specialist, in case you compromise a potentially curable cancer!*

Enquire as to whether the neck lump is painful, suggesting an inflammatory or infective process, or painless, suggesting a malignancy. The location of the lump in the neck is important in helping to construct a list of appropriate differentials.

An understanding of the anatomical triangles of the neck will help distinguish between the miscellaneous neck lumps. Although there are many potential triangles in the neck, you are only expected to know about four, particularly the anterior and posterior triangles. The key to their anatomy is identification of the sternocleidomastoid muscle, as the triangles are described in relation to this anatomical structure. Sternocleidomastoid is easiest demonstrated by asking the patient to look over to the opposite side that you are examining; you will see accentuation of the two heads of the sternocleidomastoid muscle inserting into the clavicle.

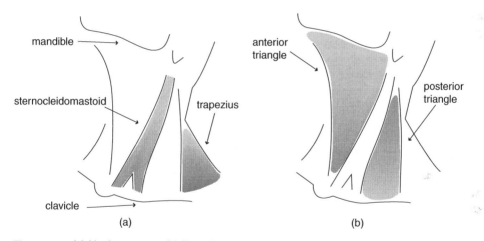

Figure 6.1: (a) Neck anatomy; (b) Triangles in the neck

The *anterior* triangle is bound by the anterior border of the sternocleidomastoid, the midline of the neck and the lower border of the mandible. The *posterior* triangle is bound by the posterior border of the sternocleidomastoid, the trapezius and the clavicle. The *submandibular* triangle is bordered by the mandible and an imaginary line between the angles of the mandible. The *parotid* triangle is an imaginary triangle just anterior to the ear at the angle of the jaw.

It is useful to classify the causes of neck lumps into the anatomical triangle in which they commonly occur. Anterior triangle lumps can be classified either anatomically or according to whether the lump exhibits pulsatility. We believe for finals the latter approach is easier.

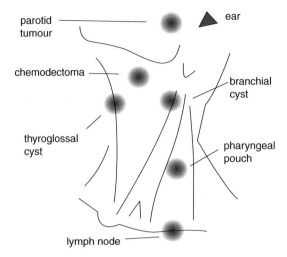

Figure 6.2: Neck lumps

Table 6.1: Differential diagnoses of neck lumps

Triangle	Pathology
Anterior	**Pulsatile** **Carotid artery aneurysm; tortuous artery.** **Carotid body tumour/chemodectoma:** Solid swelling present at bifurcation of common carotid, a bruit may be heard, usually excised due to risk of malignancy. **Non-pulsatile.** **Thyroid swellings:** Goitre, solitary thyroid nodule. **Cysts:** *Thyroglossal cyst:* Elevates with protrusion of the tongue (attachment to hyoid bone); common in those younger than 20 years and only painful if infected. *Dermoid cysts:* Epithelium-lined, congenital, benign; usually seen in those younger than 1 year. *Branchial cyst:* Fluctuant, difficult to excise as it usually forms a sinus or fistula extending backwards to the lateral pharyngeal wall; usually presents in teenage years and is painless. This has squamous cells on FNA, so must be investigated and treated urgently to distinguish from squamous cell carcinoma.
Posterior	**Subclavian aneurysm** **Pharyngeal pouch:** Presents with dysphagia and halitosis, commoner on the left and in elderly men, usually impalpable. **Cystic hygroma:** Lymphangioma, congenital lesion seen in children arising from the embryological remnants of jugular lymph sac; soft and fluctuant, varies in size and can be disfiguring. **Cervical rib:** Enlargement of costal element of C7 vertebra.

(*Continued*)

Table 6.1: Differential diagnoses of neck lumps (*Continued*)

Triangle	Pathology
Submandibular	**Salivary gland:** Tumour or stones. **Malignancy:** Primary, e.g. non-Hodgkin's lymphoma; secondary, e.g. metastasis from lip, oral cavity or facial skin cancers.
Parotid	**Inflammatory enlargement:** Viral enlargement due to mumps; bacterial secondary to an obstructing stone, sarcoid, Sjogren's syndrome. **Parotid gland tumour (Warthin's tumour; pleiomorphic adenoma)**

Remember to always consider cervical lymphadenopathy, as it is more common. A lump within the sternocleidomastoid is likely to be a sternocleidomastoid tumour. The most likely miscellaneous lumps you will encounter in finals aside from a thyroid goitre are:

Table 6.2: Examination features of miscellaneous neck lumps

Examination	Branchial cyst	Carotid body tumour	Thyroglossal cyst
Site	Anterior triangle, typically arising underneath the anterior border of the sternocleidomastoid at the upper third of the muscle	Anterior triangle at the level of the hyoid	Anterior triangle in the midline at the level of the thyroid cartilage
Consistency	Hard (can be soft) and smooth	Hard	Firm and smooth
Edge	Well-demarcated	Well-demarcated	Well-demarcated
Fluctuant	Yes	No	Yes
Fixity	Fixed to deep structures	Mobile side to side, but not up and down; overlying skin freely mobile	Fixed to deep structures (hyoid); can move side to side, but not up and down
Special features	Aspiration reveals cholesterol crystals	Pulsatile, bruit on auscultation	Moves up on tongue protrusion. Examine base of tongue for ectopic thyroid (lingual) tissue

6.2 SPECIAL NOTE ON SUBMANDIBULAR AND PAROTID TRIANGLE LUMPS

Examination of the submandibular and parotid regions requires a bimanual oral examination. You would do yourself no harm by visiting an ENT clinic, where you will gain good experience in these examinations.

Authors' Top Tip

Luckily for you, you can kill two birds with one stone, as ENT clinics often hold joint endocrine clinics for thyroid and miscellaneous neck lumps.

If there is a swelling over the parotid gland, ask the patient to open his or her mouth whilst palpating from behind, and see if the lump moves with mouth opening; this assesses whether the swelling is attached to the mandible. You will also need to look inside the mouth to see if the swelling extends into the mouth or under the tongue. This will require you to wear gloves and use a pen torch. With one hand inside the mouth and the other outside, palpate in the floor of the mouth or cheek bimanually for any lumps or stones at the ducts.

It is important to remember that for a lump in the parotid region, you must examine the seventh cranial nerve for involvement that would lead to a Bell's palsy; this would suggest malignant infiltration. On general inspection, you may see facial asymmetry characterised by a droop, loss of the nasolabial fold and an inability to close the ipsilateral eye.

6.3 THYROID

The thyroid gland is an endocrine gland that produces three hormones: thyroxine (T4), triiodothyronine (T3) and calcitonin (secreted by the parafollicular C cells). These hormones are released under the control of hormones from the hypothalamus and anterior pituitary gland (TSH). The hormones released from the thyroid gland are responsible for maintaining normal metabolism. T3 is the active form of the hormone, and T4 is converted to T3 in the periphery. The thyroid gland can become over- or under-active, resulting in a number of signs and symptoms in the individual affected.

Thyroid disease is the second-most common endocrine disorder, and disorders of thyroid function are seen more commonly in women in comparison to men.

An enlarged thyroid is known as a goitre and occurs as a result of follicular cell hyperplasia at one or more sites within the thyroid gland; although this has no correlation with the functional status of the gland, the individual can therefore be euthyroid, hypothyroid or hyperthyroid.

Authors' Top Tip

One of the most common mistakes that students make is that they palpate for the thyroid gland blindly in the neck. It is often lower than you think. This makes it important to have a good understanding of its anatomical location before you go into the examination.

The thyroid gland lies 2 cm inferior to the crest of the thyroid cartilage in the anterior part of the neck. It lies immediately under the skin and is easily accessed for inspection and palpation. The normal thyroid is easily palpable in half of all females and a quarter of the male population. The thyroid gland weighs between 15 g and 25 g, and consists of two symmetrical lateral lobes with a connecting isthmus, which lies over the second and third tracheal rings.

Often, candidates are given the instructions: 'Examine this patient's neck'. As you may not know if you are being asked to examine the thyroid or a neck lump, we have incorporated both examinations into one. It is best to start off examining the neck lump first because if you later discover it is a thyroid goitre, then you can continue with that. This seems logical, as most of your examination of a miscellaneous neck lump is inspection and so flows well with the continuity of the examination. If specifically asked to examine the thyroid, the principles for inspection are the same as for any neck lump. More often than not there are clues to the diagnosis; for example, the obvious thyroid goitre, the glass of water on the desk and the patient sitting in a chair.

With the thyroid examination, it is often safest to start with the hands. Others divide their examination into three parts: examining the lump, assessing the patient's thyroid status and checking for any associated eye signs. We will consider an all-encompassing examination.

Clinical examination

Introduction
As for any clinical encounter: (*see* Chapter 1, Section 1.3). Specifically for this case:
✔ **Position patient appropriately:** The patient is sitting on a chair, with space for you to stand behind him or her.

Authors' Top Tip

Some examiners like to challenge candidates by placing the chair against a wall; it is perfectly acceptable to ask the patient to stand and to move the chair forward, then ask the patient to sit.

✔ **Build rapport:** Inform the patient of what you are doing as you go along; remember, you are going to be feeling the patient's neck with your hand around his or her airway; this can be an intrusive examination, which may well be uncomfortable, so ask about pain as necessary.

Inspection
On general inspection, always examine from the front of the patient and from the side, as a small lump may only become visible when looking at it from the side.

The crucial point to consider is: are you dealing with a thyroid goitre or a miscellaneous neck lump? If it is obvious that you are faced with a thyroid goitre, then proceed to the hands; otherwise examine as for a lump. We will consider the situation where you are unsure.

✔ **Examine the lump**
  ▪ **Site:** This is important, as this will help decide if it's a goitre or not.
    – Which triangle is the lump in? Anterior, posterior, submandibular or parotid?
    – An anterior lump on or around the midline in the region of the thyroid cartilage is likely to be a goitre; in which case proceed as below.
  ▪ If the lump is not a goitre, then continue examining as for any lump, i.e. examine its size, shape, consistency, etc. (see Chapter 5, Lumps and bumps).

At this point, you can say to the examiner, '*I believe this is a thyroid goitre, and I would like to perform a focused thyroid examination. I would therefore like to start at the hands*'. The examiner may ask you then to go back and focus on the lump (in which case, examine the lump) or proceed with your systematic thyroid examination.

✔ **Inspect the hands**
- Do they feel warm and moist, or are they cold? Is there evidence of palmar erythema?
- Look at the nails for thyroid acropachy (clubbing), onycholysis; check their hands for vitiligo or palmar erythema, which are seen in hyperthyroidism.
- Next, ask the patient to stretch his or her arms out in front. Place a sheet of A4 paper on the hands and assess for the presence of a tremor.
- Feel the radial pulse; is the patient tachycardic or bradycardic due to propranolol use or hypothyroidism? Is there an irregular pulse (AF)?

✔ **Inspect the facies**
- **Complexion:** Peaches and cream in hypothyroidism.
- **Myxoedematous:** Thick and coarse facial features with periorbital swelling/ puffiness.
- **Eyebrows:** Loss of the outer third in hypothyroidism.

✔ **Inspect the eyes**
- Inspect for proptosis and exophthalmos (Graves' disease) from above the patient and the side. This is due to retro-orbital fat/muscle inflammation and infiltration by lymphocytes and can lead to chemosis, corneal ulcerations and opthalmoplegia.
- Look for lid retraction or lid lag. You can assess for lid lag by standing a metre away from the patient and asking him or her to fix on your finger with the eyes without moving his or her head; now move your finger in a vertical manner up and down and observe movement of the eyes and eye lids. Normally, this should occur in tandem, but in lid lag the lids will be slower than the eyes.

✔ **Inspect the mouth**
- You can look in the mouth for a lingual thyroid, where the thyroid fails to descend; it is present in the foramen caecum of the tongue.

✔ **Inspect the anterior triangle neck lump**
- **Scars:** Look for a horizontal scar at the baseline of the neck. This is also called a collar incision, or visor scar, and may indicate a previous thyroidectomy.
- **Skin changes:** Look for erythema, which can be seen in suppurative thyroiditis.
- **Tracheal deviation:** Difficult to see unless gross.
- **Tongue protrusion test:** Ask the patient to protrude the tongue; a thyroglossal cyst will rise as the tongue is protruded, while the thyroid will not.

Authors' Top Tip

If you ask the patient to tilt his or her head back, as they do so it becomes a lot easier to see this sign.

- **Swallow test:** Next, hand the patient a glass of water and ask him or her to take a mouthful and hold it. Then move the glass away and observe the neck for a swelling as you ask the patient to swallow. Do any lumps become more visible on swallowing? Do they move on swallowing? On swallowing, a goitre or thyroglossal cyst will rise due to attachment to the larynx and trachea.

✔ **Palpate the thyroid swelling**

- Palpate from behind. Warn the patient that you will be standing behind him or her and also warn before you put your hands on the neck. Before palpation, identify the anatomical boundaries, the carotid arteries, the cricoid cartilage and the suprasternal notch.
- If the carotid pulse is not palpable, this can indicate malignant thyromegaly (Berry's sign).
- Look for exophthalmos from behind, as this is seen in hyperthyroidism.
- Palpation from behind is best done with the patient's neck slightly flexed, which relaxes the sternocleidomastoid muscles.
- To identify the thyroid, locate the isthmus between the cricoid cartilage and the suprasternal notch, and palpate laterally onto the lobes of the thyroid; imagine it is in the shape of a butterfly.
- Palpate along the length of both lobes of the thyroid; they should be no longer than the length of the distal phalanx of your thumb. Comment on the consistency, volume, and temperature. Are there any abnormal swellings or nodules present? Are they localised to one lobe, or is the whole thyroid grossly swollen? Is it a smooth swelling? Or is it hard, suggestive of malignancy? Does the swelling feel multinodular? Is it tender, suggesting thyroiditis or a bleed into a cyst? Comment on the mobility of the lump; there may be tethering, as seen in malignancy. Can you feel the lower border of the thyroid? If you can't, this may suggest retrosternal extension of the gland.

Table 6.3: Consistency of the goitre

Consistency	Possible aetiology
Soft	Normal thyroid
Firm	Simple goitre
Stony, hard	Thyroid cancer, calcification, Hashimoto's
Woody	Acute thyroiditis; usually painful

- Ask the patient to repeat the swallowing test, and this time assess with palpation for the upward movement of the thyroid gland. If there is an invasive malignancy, this may tether to the surrounding structures and not move up on swallowing.
- A very large goitre that has expanded into the surrounding space may also not move when swallowing; however, most goitres move upwards on swallowing.

✔ **Assess the position of the trachea**

- Look for tracheal deviation, as seen with large retrosternal goitres.

✔ **Palpate the lymph nodes**

Systematically palpate the lymph nodes using the pulps of your index and middle fingers. Palpate both sides at the same time with the patient's head slightly flexed. Remember not to palpate over both carotid arteries simultaneously, as you may cause the patient to

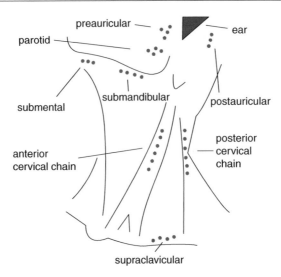

Figure 6.3: Cervical lymphatic drainage

faint! If you feel any prominent lymph nodes, comment on their position, number, size, mobility, surface and tenderness.

The technique for palpation varies and is a matter of preference.

Authors' Top Tip

We have seen some students use the so-called 'spidery technique', whereby your fingers walk along the patient's neck in the vain hope that they may feel a lymph node. We suggest you avoid this.

You are far more likely to feel a lump with the flat of your fingers as long as you are methodical in your approach and bear in mind the regional anatomical locations of the lymphatic chains. We suggest you to practice the following sequence on your colleagues in order to look slick in the OSCE:

- Palpate in front of the ears for the **preauricular** lymph nodes, moving behind the ears for the **postauricular** nodes.
- Next, follow your fingers down from the postauricular nodes to the **occipital nodes** at the base of the skull, then move onto the tonsillar nodes at the angle of the jaw and the **submandibular** nodes under the jaw on the lateral sides, moving medially to the **submental** nodes.
- Move your fingers inferiorly in front of the sternocleidomastoid muscle to palpate the **anterior superficial cervical** nodes, followed by palpation of the **supraclavicular** lymph nodes.
- The deep cervical lymph nodes are located underneath the sternocleidomastoid muscle, and you need some practice to be efficient at examining for these. The sternocleidomastoid has to be moved out of the way with the fingers of one hand and palpated with the fingers of the other; warn the patient first that this will cause them some discomfort.

Any palpable lymph nodes in the neck of a patient with a goitre are a worrying sign of metastases from a thyroid cancer. Classically, an enlarged jugulodigastric node suggests a papillary thyroid tumour metastasis.

Percussion

✔ **Check for retrosternal extension**
- Percuss over the upper part of the manubrium to assess for retrosternal extension. Its presence should be considered when there is a change in percussion note from resonant to dull.

Auscultation

✔ **Auscultate for a bruit**
- Use the diaphragm of your stethoscope to auscultate over each lobe of the thyroid to listen for a bruit, which will be heard with increased blood flow through the thyroid in hyperthyroidism/thyrotoxicosis/Graves' disease.
- When listening for this, keep in mind the presence of a carotid bruit, and do list this as one of your differentials.

Complete the examination

✔ **Further examination**
- *'To complete my examination, I would like to examine for cervical lymphadenopathy, perform a musculoskeletal examination of the neck, check for a proximal myopathy, examine the shins for pretibial myxoedema, conduct a neurological examination looking for slowly relaxing ankle reflexes and I would like to assess the quality of the patient's voice by asking her some questions'.*

Essentially you would like to further assess the patient's thyroid status and determine whether it is hyper, hypo or euthyroid. By asking the patient to cough and speak, a weak or hoarse voice suggests infiltration of the recurrent laryngeal nerve by a thyroid malignancy. If you were concerned about thyroid eye signs, you could perform a cranial nerve examination of the eyes, looking for an ophthalmoplegia.

✔ **Thank the patient**
✔ **Wash your hands**
✔ **Present your findings**

Viva questions

Q1   What is Pemberton's sign?

(Difficult Question)

- This is illustrated by facial plethora, stridor and distended neck veins as a result of obstruction.

- It occurs as a result of retrosternal extension of the goitre, leading to narrowing of the thoracic inlet and is seen when the patient is asked to raise the arms straight above his or her head.

Q2 What is Troisier's sign?
- This is the presence of an enlarged supraclavicular node in the left supraclavicular fossa.
- The node drains the thoracic duct, receiving lymph drainage from the abdomen and the left side of the thorax.
- It is enlarged as a result of metastatic deposit from a malignancy anywhere in this region.

Q3 Do you know of any goitre classification systems?

(Honours Question)

Table 6.4: WHO goitre classifications

WHO class	Clinical features
Grade 0	No goitre palpable or visible
Grade 1A	Not visible but palpable; lateral lobes smaller than the distal phalanx of the thumb
Grade 1B	Visible and palpable with neck in extended position
Grade 2	Visible with neck in normal position
Grade 3	Visible at a distance

Q4 What are the differentials of a solitary thyroid nodule?

(Difficult Question)

- A prominent nodule as part of a much larger multinodular goitre (50%).
- Benign adenoma (40%).
- Thyroid cyst (5%).
- Malignancy (5%), most commonly Papillary Thyroid Cancer.

Q5 How would you investigate this patient?
- Thyroid function tests (TFTs) and USS.

(Average Response)

Bedside tests: ECG to screen for AF, tachycardia, bradycardia.
Blood tests: TFTs, including autoantibodies.
- *In primary hypothyroidism:* Low T3 and T4 and elevated TSH.
- *In secondary hypothyroidism:* Low TSH.
- *In hyperthyroidism:* High T4 and T3, low TSH.

Imaging
- **CXR:** May demonstrate tracheal deviation or retrosternal extension in large goitres.

- **USS thyroid +/– FNAC.**
  - To determine size of the mass, although it cannot distinguish between benign or malignant.
  - Distinguishes between a solitary nodule/cyst or a prominent nodule in a multinodular goitre.
  - Distinguishes between cystic or solid nodules.
  - In a euthyroid patient, if a solitary nodule is seen, you will need to obtain a fine-needle aspiration for cytology (FNAC).

(Good Response)

Radioisotope scanning is useful for distinguishing between solitary nodules from multinodular lesions. Classically, a non-functioning nodule (cold spot) is thought to be cancerous, as opposed to a hot spot or functioning nodule. However, only 15% of cold spots are cancerous, and so most patients require FNAC to exclude cancer.

Laryngoscopy is an important preoperative investigation for those undergoing thyroid surgery to assess laryngeal nerve involvement and/or chord paralysis. This is why all preoperative thyroidectomy patients are routinely referred to ENT.

(Honours Response)

Q6 What are the causes of cervical lymphadenopathy?
  - This could be due to lymphoma, TB or infectious mononucleosis.

(Average Response)

Cervical lymphadenopathy can be either localised to the neck or part of a generalised lymphadenopathy.

Localised lymphadenopathy can be infective or neoplastic in origin:
  - *Localised infective causes include* viral, tonsillitis (jugulo-digastric nodes enlargement), mumps, TB.
  - *Localised neoplastic causes include* lymphoma.

Generalised lymphadenopathy can be infective or neoplastic in origin:
  - *Generalised infective causes include* TB, sarcoidosis, cytomegalovirus (CMV), infectious mononucleosis, HIV, toxoplasmosis.
  - *Neoplastic causes include* a primary malignancy or a secondary metastatic enlargement from some other unknown primary, e.g. thyroid cancer, lymphoma, leukaemia.

(Good Response)

'I would like to conduct a focused clinical history, a thorough examination focusing specifically on the lymphoreticular system as well as make a complete ears, nose and throat assessment. I would tailor my investigations to my findings but would generally include an FBC, an LDH and a monospot test, a CXR in those suspicious of TB or lymphoma, and a CT head and neck after discussion with an ENT specialist with a view for biopsy to exclude a head and neck malignancy'.

(Honours Response)

Q7   If your patient had a thyroglossal cyst, what else would you like to examine and why?

(Difficult Question)

- *'I would examine the base of the tongue for the presence of ectopic thyroid tissue'.*

(Good Response)

- *'Further to this* (the above), *I would request a formal USS of the neck to check for the presence of the normal thyroid gland. This is because although ectopic lingual tissue is rare, this may be the only thyroid tissue the patient has, and so if you were to excise the patient's thyroglossal cyst without first checking for a normal thyroid, this would constitute poor clinical practice'.*

(Honours Response)

This is the sort of questioning where you can gain many brownie points. In other words, do not limit yourself to what you think you can do in the examination. Say what you would do in actual clinical practise. Finals is an opportunity to test your ability to function as a good junior doctor, and so being aware of how things work in actual clinical practice and being able to communicate that in the examination will make your examiner appreciate that you will be a reliable team member, should you be his/her junior.

CHAPTER 7

Lumps and bumps: groin and testicular lumps

The examination of the groin and external genitalia forms an important part of a surgical abdominal examination and is an important examination to be competent at performing as a junior doctor. Unfortunately, many candidates get into the habit of simply stating that they would examine the hernial orifices, external genitalia and perform a digital rectal examination as part of their abdominal examination but don't actually do it in clinical practice.

Hernias are the second-most common cause of small bowel obstruction. Therefore, expect your seniors to be annoyed if you have an elderly woman presenting with abdominal pain for which no obvious cause has been identified, but you haven't yet examined her groin for hernias. You may find your consultant lifting the bed sheets off the patient to demonstrate (much to your embarrassment) a femoral hernia that could be strangulated and is the obvious cause for her symptoms. It is important to document these findings in your clinical examination. Therefore, it is no surprise that hernias are commonly examined for in surgical finals.

Often, students let themselves down because they have a poor understanding of the relevant anatomy. You should be able to describe inguinal and femoral anatomy using correct anatomical terms. We find that students tend to point or gesture towards their own groins when discussing hernia anatomy, and clearly this does not look professional. Making sure your knowledge of anatomy is sound will score you major points with the examiner.

7.1 GROIN LUMPS

There are many causes of a lump in the groin; this also includes common lumps found anywhere in the body such as sebaceous cysts, lipoma or enlarged lymph nodes. However, in finals you are most likely to be presented with a hernia.
A hernia is defined as the protrusion of a viscus or part of a viscus through a defect in the wall of its containing cavity into an abnormal position.

(Surgical Definition)

Inguinal hernias can be direct or indirect, and on occasion they can have an element of both. Up to 80% are indirect, and 20% may occur bilaterally. It is difficult to differentiate between direct and indirect inguinal hernias without taking the patient to theatre.

Indirect hernias are commonly congenital, occurring as a result of the persistence of the processus vaginalis through the deep inguinal ring. The deep inguinal ring also transmits the ilioinguinal nerve, the spermatic cord in the male and the round ligament in the female; these structures then emerge through the superficial inguinal ring. The persistence of the processus vaginalis can lead to the development of either a hydrocele in the scrotum or an indirect inguinal hernia. The sac of the hernia is composed of peritoneum, and over time this sac increases in size, as does the size of the deep ring, secondary to increasing pressure applied by the sac contents. In addition, the transversalis fascia becomes attenuated. These hernias can extend into the scrotum along with the passage of the spermatic cord, the so-called inguinoscrotal hernia.

Direct inguinal hernias present medially to the deep inguinal ring and occur secondary to weakness of the transversalis fascia; they exit through the superficial inguinal ring. Inguinal hernias are more common in males, whereas femoral hernias are relatively more common in females, although a hernia is more likely to be inguinal in origin even when present in a female, as inguinal hernias overall are far more common than femoral in either sex.

Femoral hernias exit with the femoral vessels into the femoral canal and can be confused with inguinal hernias. Femoral hernias are at high risk of strangulation due to the narrow neck of the femoral canal, and as a result if identified should be repaired electively at the earliest given opportunity. This is also the reason why you are unlikely to see such a case in finals. If you are unsure of the diagnosis in the examination, the odds are that it is likely to be an inguinal hernia, of which the indirect type is the commonest.

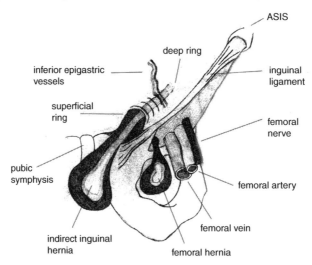

Figure 7.1: Anatomy of the groin

Clinical examination

Introduction

As for any clinical encounter (*see* Chapter 1, Principles of a clinical encounter). Specifically for this case:

✔ **Ask for a chaperone:** Turn to the examiner, and ask for a chaperone.
✔ **Build rapport:** Inform patient of what you are doing as you go along; remember that you are going to be feeling the patient's groin; this is an intimate and intrusive examination that may be uncomfortable for the patient, so ask about pain as necessary.

Inspection

This should be done with the patient standing initially, as the hernia can reduce when lying supine but becomes more obvious when standing. Remember to examine both sides. Ideally you should be sitting on a stool in front of the patient, looking from both the front and the side of the patient.
✔ **Observe with the patient standing**
  ▪ **Scars:** Are there any from previous hernia operations?
  ▪ **Lumps:** Are they above or below the skin crease? If there is a lump, describe as you would for any lump; include site, size, etc. (*see* Chapter 5, Lumps and bumps) Specifically check to see if this lump extends into the scrotum.
  ▪ If there is no obvious lump, ask the patient to cough or perform a Valsalva manoeuvre; this may accentuate any hernias, if present.

Palpation

Examine both sides, using your right hand to examine from the right side and your left hand to examine the left.
✔ **Palpate the lump**
  ▪ Describe as you would any lump (*see* Chapter 5, Lumps and bumps); specifically see if the lump is tender.
  ▪ If the mass is a hernia and is tender to touch, this may suggest obstruction or ischaemia.
✔ **Check for a cough impulse**
  ▪ Apply gentle pressure over the lump and ask the patient to cough.
  ▪ If the lump expands on coughing, this is said to be a positive test, suggesting a hernia or saphena varix.

Remember that with an expansile mass, your fingers will displace laterally when you place one finger on either side of the lump.
  At this point, you may ask the patient to now lie supine on the examining couch.
✔ **Define the anatomy**
  ▪ **Mark your anatomical landmarks:** Locate the ASIS and the pubic tubercle; demonstrate that the inguinal ligament runs between these two points; locate the deep ring which is found at the midpoint of the inguinal ligament.

Authors' Top Tip

This initial approach not only orientates you but also tells the examiner you are well versed in inguinal and femoral hernia anatomy. Expect to be questioned about the relevant anatomy in your viva.

The pubic tubercle is the most laterally palpable part of the pubic crest and is 1.5 cm lateral to the pubic symphysis.

✔ **Distinguish between a femoral and inguinal hernia**
  ■ **Reduce the hernia:** If you attempt to reduce the hernia yourself, you risk hurting the patient. Often the patient is an expert at doing this. It is perfectly acceptable to ask the patient if the hernia is reducible and if they could kindly push it back in themselves for you to see.
  ■ With one hand on the ASIS and the other over the pubic tubercle, identify the anatomical location of the hernia in relation to the pubic tubercle. The pubic tubercle approximates the **superficial ring** (the most lateral end of the ring).
    – **Above and medial:** Inguinal.
    – **Below and lateral:** Femoral.

You can ask the patient to cough to accentuate the lump.

At this point, your findings will determine how you carry on with your examination. As you are more likely to get an inguinal hernia in the examination, we will continue as for an inguinal hernia examination.

✔ **Distinguish between a direct and indirect inguinal hernia**
  ■ **Reduce the hernia:** Ask the patient to do this.
  ■ **Redefine anatomy:** Locate the **deep ring** and place two fingers over it. This is done in an attempt to control the hernia.
    – The **deep ring** is found at the 'midpoint of the inguinal ligament.'
    – This is a point halfway between the ASIS and the pubic tubercle.

Authors' Top Tip

Do not confuse this with the term 'mid-inguinal point', which is a point halfway between the ASIS and the pubic symphysis. This is the site of the femoral artery.

Note that the deep ring is also known as the internal ring.
  ■ **Deep ring occlusion test:** Ask the patient to cough, and see if the hernia pops out.
    – **Hernia controlled:** Indirect inguinal hernia.
    – **Hernia not controlled:** Direct inguinal hernia.

Of course, in actual clinical practice this test is unreliable. For the purpose of finals, the only way to be sure is in theatre, when you can compare the position of the hernia to the inferior epigastric vessels intraoperatively (*see* Viva Q6).

✔ **Examine the scrotum**
  ■ This involves a standard examination (*see* Chapter 7, Section 7.2 Testicular Lumps).
  ■ Specifically consider undescended testicles, and in the case of a lump, check for extension of the hernia into the scrotum.

A large, indirect, inguinal hernia extending into the scrotum may be mistaken for a hydrocele. You can differentiate the two by shining a light into the lump in the dark and assessing for the presence of transilluminance, which would suggest a hydrocele.

Percussion
✔ Percuss over the hernia
- **Hyper-resonant:** Bowel contents.
- **Dull:** More likely to represent omentum or fat in the hernia sac.

Auscultation
✔ Auscultate over the hernia
- If you suspect bowel contents, listen for audible bowel sounds; if they are absent, it suggests strangulation.

Complete the examination
✔ Examine the opposite side
- If you have not already done so, then you must examine the opposite groin.

It is not enough to say that you will examine the opposite groin; you must actually begin to examine the opposite groin. Remember, 20% of inguinal hernias are bilateral. The examiner will most likely be happy that you have considered this and will usually stop you.

✔ Further examination
- *'To complete my examination, I would like to examine the abdomen and testicles'.*
✔ Thank the patient
✔ Wash your hands
✔ Present your findings, e.g.:

'On examination, there is a 4 by 4 cm lump in the right groin; the lump is soft, painless and reducible. It lies above and medial to the pubic tubercle and is controlled by direct pressure over the deep ring. This is most likely to be an indirect inguinal hernia'.

Percussion and auscultation add very little to your examination but have been presented for completeness.

Authors' Top Tip

You may find many definitions of the anatomical site of the deep ring, and these often fluster candidates. It is sufficient to know that the deep ring is at the midpoint of the inguinal ligament.

Viva questions

Q1 What are the borders of the femoral canal?
- Inguinal ligament, pectineal ligament, femoral vein and lacunar ligament.

(Average Response)

- **Anterior border:** Inguinal ligament.
- **Posterior border:** Pectineal ligament.
- **Lateral border:** Femoral vein.
- **Medial border:** Lacunar ligament.

(Good Response)

The femoral canal contains fatty tissues, lymphatic vessels and the deep inguinal lymph node (the nodes of Cloquet).

Q2 What are the borders of the femoral triangle?
- The inguinal ligament, the medial border of sartorius and the adductor longus.
- The femoral triangle abuts Hunter's canal from above.
- The floor is made up of psoas, pectineus and adductor longus.

(Good Response)

Authors' Top Tip

A good response to any question asking for anatomical borders will always try to be as accurate as possible, with candidates not only identifying the structures that make up the borders but also the position of those borders.

The femoral triangle contains the femoral vessels and nerve. Hunter's canal contains the femoral artery, the femoral vein and the saphenous nerve. The canal also contains 'the nerve to vastus Medialis'. This is a site of anatomic narrowing, commonly resulting in occlusive vascular disease'.

Q3 What are the borders of the inguinal canal?
- **Superior:** Conjoint tendon.
- **Inferior:** Inguinal ligament.
- **Anterior:** External oblique aponeurosis.
- **Posterior:** Transversalis fascia.

(Good Response)

- The inguinal canal is an oblique, 4-cm long intermuscular slit that is bordered **posteriorly** by transversalis fascia, which is reinforced by the conjoint tendon medially.
- Its **anterior border** is external oblique aponeurosis, which is reinforced laterally by the internal oblique.
- **Inferiorly** a floor is formed, mostly by the inguinal ligament laterally but also by the lacunar ligament medially.
- **Superiorly** a roof is formed by the arching fibres of the transversus abdominis muscle (the lateral half) and the internal oblique muscle (the lateral two thirds), which fuse together into an aponeurosis to form the conjoint tendon medially and act to strengthen the posterior wall as well.

(Honours Response)

The inguinal canal runs from the deep ring to the superficial ring and is approximately 4- to 6-cm long. It transports the spermatic cord in men, the round ligament in women, and the ilioinguinal nerve.

The superficial ring is a V-shaped slit in the external oblique aponeurosis that allows the contents of the canal to exit, into e.g. the scrotum. You may be able to invaginate a lump in the scrotum back to the superficial ring and discover an inguinoscrotal hernia.

Q4 What is the differential diagnosis of a lump in the groin?

(Difficult Question)

This question is best answered by considering the anatomical structures in the groin. From superficial to deep, they are:

- **Skin and subcutaneous tissues:** Sebaceous cyst, lipoma.
- **Muscle:** Psoas abscess.
- **Hernia:** Femoral or inguinal.
- **Vein:** Saphena varix (varicosity at the sapheno-femoral junction, which usually disappears on lying down).
- **Artery:** Femoral artery aneurysm, pseudoaneurysm (the latter is more common).
- **Lymph nodes:** Inguinal lymphadenopathy.
- **Ectopic structures:** Undescended or maldescended testes (palpate the scrotum to confirm the absence of testicle); renal transplant in the RIF (although usually not as far down in the groin).

It is important to remember that if you find inguinal lymphadenopathy, tell the examiner that you will check that this is not part of a generalised lymphadenopathy. Lymphoma is a diagnosis you do not wish to miss, so be sure to examine for hepatosplenomegaly and take a careful history for fever, night sweats and weight loss. Testicular malignancies leading to inguinal lymphadenopathy are unusual; typically lymphatic spread is to the aortic and retroperitoneal lymph nodes, which of course would be difficult or nearly impossible to feel on clinical examination. It is the scrotum that drains to the superficial inguinal lymph nodes.

Q5 How would you investigate a hernia?

(Difficult Question)

- Hernias are diagnosed primarily on history and clinical examination alone; rarely are additional tests performed.
- The gold standard test is a herniography. This is where an intra-peritoneal injection of water soluble contrast is administered, and the patient is screened for a hernial sac while standing.
- Today, USS of groin and scrotum is used routinely as needed for suspected groin hernias.

Q6 How would you differentiate an indirect from direct inguinal hernia?
- The gold standard method is intraoperatively in theatres by assessing the hernia with respect to the inferior epigastric vessels.

- These vessels form part of Hesselbach's triangle, which can be defined intraoperatively by its three borders, bounded:
    - *Medially* by rectus abdominis.
    - *Inferiorly* by inguinal ligament.
    - *Superiorly* and laterally by the inferior epigastric vessels.
- The indirect hernial defect is the superficial ring, which is lateral to the inferior epigastrics.
- A direct hernial defect tends to go through Hesselbach's triangle, which is medial to the inferior epigastrics.
- This is the reason for the common phrase, 'With respect to the inferior epigastric vessels', i.e. medial to the vessels is a direct inguinal hernia, and lateral is indirect.

(Good Response)

Q7   What are the principles of hernia repair?

(Difficult Question)

- *'Herniorrhaphy can be performed open or laparoscopically.*
- *Open repairs can be done under general, regional or even local anaesthetic.*
- *Surgical repair involves the following four general principles: define the anatomy, inspect and excise the hernial sac, close the defect and confirm the repair is tension free'.*

In hernioplasty, the defect is reinforced with a prosthetic mesh. In a herniotomy, the hernial sac is completely excised; this is typically performed in children. There are many methods for repairing a hernia, but for undergraduate purposes you will not be expected to know these, let alone their various eponymous names. Being aware of the above four principles will allow you to have an intelligent discussion with the examiner.

7.2   TESTICULAR LUMPS

In our experience, being asked to examine a scrotum usually strikes fear into the eyes of candidates. This is because a scrotal examination isn't usually something that students practice and adequately prepare. This is a shame, as the examination is actually very straightforward, with a limited variety of possible cases. It is very easy to spot the candidate who is making up the examination as he or she goes along.

Examiner's Anecdote

'I couldn't believe she started to percuss the scrotum! I could see the look of horror on the patient's face!'

You are most likely to see a hydrocele in finals; however, do not be fooled by an inguino-scrotal hernia. Although you will not be expected to have a detailed knowledge of urology, being able to examine a scrotum confidently will stand you in good stead.

Often, students ask us if it is necessary to wear gloves when examining in finals. The opinion on this differs. We remember one of our general surgical consultants (who was also a finals examiner) who said that he would expect you not to wear gloves. His reasoning was that you don't generally wear gloves when examining a patient, unless for infection control purposes, and thus it seems unprofessional. However, having recently finished a urology post and spoken to countless urology consultants who frequently examine in finals, they all advised to wear gloves. If available, use gloves; if not, then you may have to soldier on. However, please be sure to wash your hands before starting the examination and before proceeding to the next case; both your patients and examiners will greatly appreciate it!

Also, listen carefully to the instructions; you may be told to examine the groin, where in fact the testicles are the site of pathology.

As this is an intimate examination, it is crucial you request a chaperone, even if you are a male candidate. Make sure your hands are not too cold, as this will cause involuntary contraction of the dartos muscle and make it difficult to examine the scrotal contents (cremasteric reflex).

Clinical examination

Introduction
As for any clinical encounter (*see* Chapter 1, Principles of a clinical encounter). Specifically for this case:
✔ Ask for a chaperone

Inspection
This should be done with the patient supine initially, then ask the patient to stand, as you don't want to miss a varicocele. You may need to lift the scrotum with your hand to visually inspect its posterior aspect.
✔ Check for any obvious abnormalities:
  ▪ **Colour:** Erythema, suggestive of inflammation; bruising, suggestive of trauma.
  ▪ **Scars:** Over the median raphe, but usually difficult to see. You may see a hernia scar.
  ▪ **Symmetry:** The left testicle usually hangs slightly lower than the right.
  ▪ **Size:** Any obvious atrophy or swellings.
  ▪ **Abnormal lie:** Bell clapper deformity, as seen in torsion (extremely unlikely in the examination).
  ▪ **Swellings:** Scrotal, inguinal, whether it is unilateral/bilateral, hydrocele, varicocele (seen best on standing).

Palpation
✔ Check for a hernia
  ▪ **Examine as above for a hernia, with extension into the scrotum.**

This is important to do first, as the case may have simply been an inguinoscrotal hernia. The examiner may ask you to skip this if the pathology is obviously scrotal in origin.

✔ **Palpate each testicle**
Palpate each individual testis between your thumb and forefinger gently for:
- **Consistency:** There is normally a rubbery texture. Are there any lumps? Is it soft or hard? Is it tender?
- **Absence:** Are both testicles present?
- **Size:** Are the testes the same size? They are normally 4 by 2 cm.
- **Swelling:** If there is a very large swelling, consider a hydrocele.

✔ **Examine any swellings**
If there is a swelling present, examine for the following:
- **Separate:** Is the lump separate from the testicle? This distinguishes between scrotal pathology and a hernia extending from the groin.
- **Extension:** Can you get above the lump, i.e. is it extending from the superficial ring? If you can't get above the lump, then this is probably an inguino-scrotal hernia; examine as above for a hernia.
- **Transilluminable:** Is it transilluminable? Shine a torch light on the scrotal mass in a darkened environment to distinguish between fluid and solid mass. Often in the examination, it is enough to cast a shadow over the scrotum with your free hand whilst you transilluminate with the other.

There are a plethora of tips from seniors regarding how to transilluminate a testicular swelling, ranging from a modified Smarties box to other ingenious tricks of the trade. However, we suggest you keep things simple. Have a dedicated, preferably disposable, pen torch with you in the examination and simply transilluminate by placing the end of the torch close to the scrotum. Be careful not to keep the torch there too long, as a localised heat source may cause pain to the patient! Also, remember to dispose of or clean the torch for the next case, as you do not want to shine the same torch into a patient's mouth!

✔ **Palpate the epididymis and spermatic cord**
- The epididymis is located posteriorly and lateral to the testicle lying longitudinally; it is smooth and soft. The spermatic cord feels like pliable tubing.
- Is it tender or thickened, as seen in epididymo-orchitis?

✔ **Palpate for lymph nodes in the inguinal region**
- Check for inguinal lymphadenopathy.

Complete the examination

✔ **Further examination**
- *'To complete my examination, I would like to examine the abdomen and groin'.*

✔ **Thank the patient**

✔ **Wash your hands**

✔ **Present your findings**

Please note there is no percussion and auscultation in a general scrotal examination. The key to the examination is to distinguish between an inguinoscrotal hernia and a true scrotal pathology. Once you are certain this case is scrotal, then the following are the most likely causes:

Table 7.1: Possible causes

Examination	Hydrocele	Varicocele	Epididymal cyst	Testicular mass
Separate lump	Unable to separate from testis	Separate from testis	Separate from testis (in the epididymis)	Unable to separate from testis
Consistency	Firm or tense	'Bag of worms'	Firm	Hard, nodular
Transilluminable	Yes	No	Yes (in large cysts)	No
Extension	Can get above the mass	Can get above the mass	Can get above the mass	Can get above the mass
Special features	Can be very large, leading to a grossly swollen testicle	Disappears on lying flat (unless sinister); palpable cough impulse; usually left sided	Often multiple. If it contains sperm (due to a complication of vasectomy), it will not transilluminate. Can be painful.	Non-tender; there may be an associated hydrocele

Viva questions

Q1   If I told you that a patient's varicocele developed rapidly over the last few weeks, what pathology would you consider?

(Difficult Question)

- *'In an older patient, I would consider the possibility of retroperitoneal disease, specifically external compression of the left renal vein due to a mass, possibly a renal cell carcinoma'.*

Varicoceles are dilated tortuous veins of the pampiniform plexus. A rapid onset, particularly one that does not disappear on lying down, suggests sinister pathology. Varicoceles typically affect the left testicle as the left testicular vein is longer and often lacks a terminal valve, plus the draining left renal vein is vulnerable to external compression by the colon (or in some cases a renal mass). It can lead to infertility later in life. Treatment is embolisation of the testicular vein.

Q2   How would you treat a hydrocele?

(Difficult Question)

Conservative measures

- Reassurance and observation for small hydroceles, or those in whom a tumour has been excluded.
- Aspiration of fluid for symptom relief in large hydroceles, but this isn't effective, as the fluid tends to re-accumulate and there is a risk of introducing infection into the hydrocele.

Current practice is moving away from aspiration, with some urologists making it an absolute contraindication unless you can confidently exclude an underlying testicular malignancy because aspiration can lead to tumour seeding through the tract to the scrotal skin.

Surgical measures

- There are a number of eponymously named procedures; it is sufficient to know that there are surgical options available, although there is a high recurrence rate.

A hydrocele is an abnormal accumulation of fluid in the tunica vaginalis. Fluid can accumulate due to a number of reasons: a hydrocele can be secondary to a testicular tumour, orchitis or trauma. The key feature to remember for finals is that hydroceles should always be scanned with a USS testes; this is because there may be an underlying testicular tumour that would be difficult to feel if the hydrocele is particularly large or tense.

CHAPTER 8

Surgical emergencies

8.1 PRINCIPLES OF SURGICAL EMERGENCIES

Management of emergencies forms the basis of most of the viva discussions that you will have in surgical finals. The examiner is not, however, assessing your understanding of detailed operative management of a given emergency. It is the underlying principles central to surgical management that they are interested. The examiner is trying to assess whether you will be a safe junior doctor. It is therefore essential that you call for help early, as this is likely to form a part of the mark scheme. However, be careful: candidates assume that calling for help absolves them of any other management responsibilities. This is not true; very often in actual clinical practice your senior is scrubbed up in theatre with an emergency case and cannot come to your aid immediately. You therefore need to be able to resuscitate the patient whilst awaiting senior review. You need to be logical, calm and methodical in your approach to an emergency. And so emergency treatment will always start with the well-known Airway (A), Breathing (B) and Circulation (C) model taught in medical schools.

This initial assessment is the cornerstone of surgical and medical emergency management and should be ingrained into your mind for the remainder of your career. You cannot expect the cavalry to arrive when you have not even done the basics. Many times we have come onto the scene when a junior has called for help only to find that the patient wasn't on supplemental oxygen, there was no intravenous access gained and there had been no attempt to fluid resuscitate the patient. This is not acceptable, and being a junior does not excuse you from having a thorough understanding of the initial assessment.

Examiner's Anecdote

'When he said, "I would do A,B,C's innit!" I asked him to stop and tell me what exactly he would do; he only knew what the acronym stood for. I was not impressed'.

The initial assessment allows you to simultaneously perform a focused clinical examination and treat any abnormalities before moving onto the next system. As the A, B, C model prioritises the recognition and treatment of illness in order of its relative threat to life, you cannot, e.g. proceed from B to C unless you have managed or treated any problems you have found in B.

Authors' Top Tip

*Do not say in the exam that you would refer to the surgical team, as you **are** the surgical team. Although you would not be expected to perform a burr hole in a patient with an extra-dural haematoma, you should at the very least be aware of the treatment options available.*

Below, we describe a schema to use whenever you are asked about the management of any surgical emergency. Note that only in the case of emergencies does the term 'management' not require you to take a history and perform a clinical examination. In actual clinical practise, however, this is done simultaneously, and the top students put this across to the examiner in their discussion. Irrespective of the underlying diagnosis, the initial management is the same for all patients, and any collaborating history can be taken once the patient has been stabilised.

Initial assessment of a surgical emergency

✔ **Recognition of emergency**
  ▪ Examiners want you to appreciate the urgency of the treatment and want to see this in your answer.
  ▪ We suggest to simply state, *'This is a surgical emergency. I will resuscitate the patient by...'*
✔ **Assess the airway (A)**
  ▪ **Give supplemental oxygen:** Always give the patient high-flow oxygen via a non-rebreather bag.
  ▪ **Assess patency:** Ask the patient a question; if he or she responds, then the airway is maintained. If not, then:
    – **Assess for evidence of airway compromise:** Look in the oral cavity for anything blocking the airway, such as blood or vomitus, and suction this using a Yankauer suction. Listen for stridor, which suggests impending airway compromise.
    – **Establish a patent airway:** Do this using the following airway manoeuvres:
      ❑ **Simple manoeuvres:** Jaw thrust, chin lift; remove any foreign bodies.
      ❑ **Airway adjuncts:** If the patient cannot maintain the airway, then use simple airway adjuncts, such as an oropharyngeal airway (Guedel) or a nasopharyngeal airway.
      ❑ **Secure/definitive airway:** If the patient's GCS is <8, or you are worried the patient may lose his or her airway for any reason, you will need expert help to insert a definitive airway. This can be in the form of orotracheal intubation, e.g. endotracheal tube, or a surgical airway, e.g. cricothyroidotomy.

A definitive airway is one where a cuffed tube is secured in the trachea, ensuring patency.

(Surgical Definition)

✔ **Check the Breathing (B)**
- **Monitoring:** Attach a saturation probe to assess the level of oxygen saturation, although ideally you would perform an ABG to determine the actual oxygen saturation in the blood.
- **Inspection:** Does the patient look cyanosed, suggesting imminent respiratory arrest? Assess the respiratory rate; an increased respiratory rate >20 is a sensitive sign of disease. Look for equal chest wall expansion and/or any distended neck veins in case the patient has a pneumothorax; paradoxical chest wall movement suggests evidence of a flail chest.
- **Palpation:** Assess for tracheal deviation; percuss the chest wall for hyperresonance in a pneumothorax or dullness in postoperative basal atelectasis or a haemothorax.
- **Auscultate:** Listen to breath sounds for lung pathology.

The purpose of assessing breathing is to ensure adequate ventilation.

✔ **Assess Circulation (C)**
- **Assess level of shock:** Is the patient cool and clammy? Check capillary refill time, which is normally <3 seconds.
- **Monitoring:** Attach the patient to a monitor and check vital signs, i.e. HR and BP.
- **Obtain IV access:** Insert two large-bore cannulae (grey or brown); one into each antecubital fossa. Take this opportunity to take bloods for further investigation.
- **Resuscitation fluids:** If the patient is haemodynamically unstable, start resuscitating using intravenous fluids, e.g. normal saline.
- **Additional monitoring:** Consider inserting a urinary catheter and/or central line to help gauge fluid resuscitation and response.

Hypovolaemia should be the first condition you consider in a surgical patient who is haemodynamically unstable. Resuscitation fluid that you can use can be crystalloids, colloids or blood (*see* Chapter 11, Surgical instruments: Case 2).

✔ **Assess Disability (D)**
Assess the patient's neurological status, pupil size and BM glucose levels.
- **Neurological status:** This can be estimated using the GCS score; or the Alert, Verbal response, response to Pain, Unresponsive (AVPU).
- **Pupils:** Check to detect cases of opiate overdose (bilateral pinpoint pupils), or for a blown pupil (unilaterally dilated pupil) in a space-occupying lesion such as a subdural or extradural haematoma.
- **BM glucose:** Should be checked in case the neurological status is secondary to blood glucose derangement, which is easily amenable to treatment.

✔ **Assess Environment (E)**
- Expose the patient, as this may help in your diagnosis.
- For example, the hypotensive patient who is bleeding per rectum may have lost blood that is being hidden by the bed sheets.
- From a surgical point of view, this is probably the best opportunity to assess the abdomen, e.g. for a pulsatile/expansile mass.

✔ **Assess response to initial measures**
- If something has changed, whether in breathing or circulation, always start from the beginning again and reassess the patient's A, B and C's.
- Likewise, if the patient is showing signs of improvement, reassess again; there may have been a hidden pathology that can now be unmasked.

Authors' Top Tip

If the examiner is probing you for an answer and you are unsure what to do, the best reply is to say that you will go back and reassess the patient's A, B and C's to see if there is anything you have missed. This shows you are being systematic in your approach and will not miss out on any life-threatening injuries.

✔ **Emergency investigations**
Investigations can be done to help aid your diagnosis, e.g. requesting a serum amylase in a patient with an acute abdomen. These are divided into:
- **Simple bedside tests:** ECG, pregnancy test, BM glucose.
- **Blood tests:** FBC, U&Es, etc.; ABG as appropriate (especially if critically ill).
- **Imaging:** Erect CXR; CT abdomen.
- **Specialist investigations:** These depend on your differentials.

If the patient is still unstable and requires definitive surgical treatment, then you must forgo non-essential investigations, e.g. the ruptured AAA should never have a CT abdomen, as the patient will arrest in the scanner!

Examiner's Anecdote

'The patient clearly had a ruptured AAA, and after having informed the candidate that the patient was going to the CT scanner, he replied by saying that he would assess the patient when coming back. I told him, "I don't think your patient will come back!" In clear-cut cases where patients need immediate operative treatment, investigations are not necessary; they should be taken straight to theatre. Don't forget the exploratory laparotomy is an investigation in its own right'.

✔ **Call for senior help and advice**
- Note that at this stage, you are calling for senior help and advice once the patient is stabilised or informing your senior of an unstable patient who requires immediate operative treatment.

In actual clinical practice, once your seniors have arrived, they may refer the patient or ask you to refer to other specialities for advice, e.g. intensive treatment unit (ITU).

Authors' Top Tip

If the patient who has deteriorated is currently an inpatient, then a courtesy call is commonly made to the patient's own consultant, informing him or her of recent events even if the consultant is not on call with you. Rest assured that consultants will be annoyed the following morning if they have not been informed of a sick patient under their care.

✔ Definitive treatment
- This can be either conservative, medical or surgical.
- If you suspect the patient will require immediate surgical treatment, then use your initiative and state that you will book an emergency theatre slot. Inform the theatre nurse coordinator and the on-call anaesthetist, then organise consent from the patient.

Completion

The examiner may ask you further questions regarding the original diagnosis.

Authors' Top Tip

Do not play 'tennis' with the examiner by continually asking for further information, with the examiner replying by telling you it is normal or negative. The examiner will usually give you enough information at the beginning and will offer laboratory values as needed in your discussion. The examiner is not trying to trick you; neither is he holding out. He is trying to pass you.

As the initial management for any surgical emergency is essentially the same, for purposes of clarity we have given an example of a thorough viva discussion in the first case only.

Case 1: Acute pancreatitis

Instructions: This 35-year-old woman has complained of right upper quadrant pain. Her serum amylase is 3 500. How would you manage her?

Viva discussion

- **Recognise urgency:** *'This is a surgical emergency'.*
- **Initial resuscitation:** *'I would resuscitate the patient, ensuring the patient's airway is patent with access to high-flow supplemental oxygen. I would then ensure the patient is breathing adequately. I will address the circulation by inserting two large-bore cannulae, one into each antecubital fossa, whilst taking blood for pancreatic severity assessment at the same time. I would begin the patient on aggressive fluid resuscitation, as the patient is likely to have suffered significant third-space loss'.*
- **Additional monitoring:** *'To accurately guide fluid replacement, I would like to assess the patient's volume status through clinical examination, the patient's vital signs and urine output. As such, the patient will need to be catheterised and a strict fluid balance chart documented in order to maintain a positive balance'.*
- **Call for help:** *'At this point, I would call for senior help and advice. After discussion with a senior colleague, I would like to consider the need for a CVP line to accurately guide fluid replacement'.*
- **Assess severity:** *'I would then like to assess the severity of this pancreatitis attack, as this will help determine the level of care the patient requires, particularly the need for an HDU bed. Using the modified Glasgow severity score, I would perform an arterial blood gas analysis on air to check for type one respiratory failure with a pO2 of <8, as this would suggest ARDS. I would also check for*

a metabolic acidosis and serum lactate levels, as this gives an indication of the level of shock. Other specific tests I would request include glucose levels to check for hyperglycaemia, as the patient may need an insulin sliding scale, plus serum calcium levels and particularly a CRP, as this helps to monitor and guide treatment. Other investigations I would like to request include a plain abdominal radiograph to check for calcified gallstones as a possible cause, and a CXR to check for signs of ARDS'.

- **Definitive treatment:**
  - *'I would keep the patient NBM, consider nutritional support (enteral, or parenteral in severe cases) and ensure good pain relief in the form of a PCA through a dedicated line'.*
  - *'I would request a USS to check for stones in the biliary tree and any bile duct dilatation. If there is any bile duct dilatation, I would speak to a senior colleague with regards to the need for an ERCP +/– sphincterotomy at a later suitable time'.*
  - *'Eventually the patient will require an abdominal CT with pancreatic protocol to check for pancreatic necrosis. If this shows necrosis, I would discuss with my seniors the need for a radiological-guided aspiration of peripancreatic fluid to check for an infected necrosis +/– intravenous antibiotics and surgical debridement via a necrosectomy, which is indicated when the pancreas is 70% necrotic'.*
  - *'Eventually the patient will require a cholecystectomy if the cause of the attack has been gallstones. Some centres prefer to wait 6 weeks after recovery, while others elect for same-stay surgery'.*

(Honours Response)

Completion

You can see that by following a methodical approach, you will have been talking to the examiner for only a few minutes and scoring many points!

Viva questions

Q1 What are the causes of pancreatitis?

Remember the famous acronym, 'GET SMASHED':

- **G:** Gallstones (by far the most common cause of pancreatitis in the United Kingdom).
- **E:** Ethanol (the second-most common cause).
- **T:** Trauma.
- **S:** Steroids.
- **M:** Mumps.
- **A:** Autoimmune diseases.
- **S:** Scorpion bites.

- **H:** Hyperlipidaemia, hypercalcaemia.
- **E:** ERCP.
- **D:** Drugs, e.g. thiazide diuretics.

Q2 What fluids would you give?

(Difficult Question)

- *'A crystalloid solution, such as Hartmann's, or normal saline'.*

(Average Response)

- *'As the patient has suffered significant third space loss, I would like to use an isotonic crystalloid solution, such as Hartmann's, as this will replace ECF loss'.*

(Good Response)

- *'The constituent ions of Hartmann's solution are very similar to the ECF compartment. As pancreatitis leads to fluid loss, which is mainly ECF, replacing with an isotonic crystalloid seems the logical choice'.*

(Honours Response)

Q3 How much fluid would you give?
- *'Patients should receive maintenance fluids plus additional losses. As this patient is likely to have suffered significant third space loss, it would not be unusual to give 6 L or more in 1 day'.*

(Average Response)

- *'However, I would first need to assess the patient's volume status and guide fluid replacement according to that'.*
- *'Empirically, I would give 1 L stat, followed by another 1 L over the first hour, then another 1 L over the subsequent 2 hours, another over the next 3 hours and then 6 hourly thereafter. This would be guided by the fluid balance chart, which should be strictly kept'.*

(Good Response)

Q4 How would you assess the severity of the attack?

(Difficult Question)

- Use the Glasgow Prognostic Score (in the first 48 hours):
    - **P:** Arterial pO_2 <8 kPa.
    - **A:** Age >55 years.
    - **N:** Neutrophils >15 × 10^9/L.
    - **C:** Calcium <2 mmol/L.
    - **R:** Raised urea >16 mmol/L.
    - **E:** Elevated enzymes AST > 125 or LDH > 600 IU.
    - **A:** Albumin <32 g/L.
    - **S:** Sugar (i.e. glucose) >10 mmol/L.

- Score of 1: mild, 2: moderate; 3: severe.
- A score of '3' or more is an indication for management in the HDU.
- Independent from the above variables, a CRP > 150 constitutes a severe attack.

Authors' Top Tip

There are many other severity scores for pancreatitis, and some for specific aetiologies. We suggest you learn the one above, as it is the easiest to remember.

Q5 What are the types of pancreatitis?
- Oedematous (most common), haemorrhagic (look for Grey Turner's or Cullen's signs) and necrotising pancreatitis.

Q6 Would you start antibiotics?

(Difficult Question)

- *'The use of antibiotics in pancreatitis is controversial. However, in this case I would follow trust protocol with regards to the use of antibiotics'.*
- *'In cases of doubt or an infected pancreatic necrosis, I would discuss with the on-call microbiologist as well as with my seniors with regards to the need for antibiotics in accordance with the patient's clinical condition'.*

Q7 What diagnosis would you consider if a patient had a persistently raised amylase?

(Honours Question)

- A pancreatic pseudocyst is the likely cause.
- This commonly occurs in pancreatitis due to alcohol and is confirmed on CT scan.
- Those <6 cm in size resolve within 6 weeks; larger ones may need to be percutaneously drained under radiological guidance.

Case 2: Upper GI bleed

Instructions: This man has presented with haematemesis. How would you manage him?

Key features to mention:

Viva discussion
- **Recognise urgency.**
- **Initial resuscitation:** *See above* and assess level of hypovolaemic shock.

- **Emergency investigations:** FBC, U&E (raised urea suggests recent GI bleeding), LFT, amylase, clotting, CX at least 4 U of blood.
- **Additional monitoring:** CVP line and catheter to accurately guide resuscitation.
- **Call for help:** *'After discussion with a senior colleague, I would like to consider the need for an emergency OGD in the unstable patient'.*
- **Assess severity:** Rockall score (*see below*).
- **Definitive treatment:**
  - *Consider* resuscitation with blood if still hypotensive.
  - *PPI* in those with known peptic ulcer disease.
  - *Emergency* OGD to identify source of bleeding and treat.
  - *Sengstaken-Blakemore tube* as a holding manoeuvre if there is massive bleeding and the patient is still awaiting definitive treatment.
  - *Surgery* if uncontrolled bleeding, re-bleeding, recurrent hypotension or the bleeding site is not identified at OGD.

Completion

Never forget to CX blood; this is why it is so important to stick to a methodical routine when managing an acutely unwell surgical patient. Always follow the initial resuscitation measures we have discussed above, and you will be fine.

Authors' Top Tip

We once knew a consultant who stated that if a candidate forgot to mention he would insert nothing less than a large-bore cannula in the antecubital fossa in the above case, the consultant would fail the candidate! Ensure you do not make the same mistake.

Viva questions

Q1 What are the causes of an upper GI bleed?
- Duodenal ulcer (the most common).
- Gastritis, oesophageal varices.
- Mallory-Weiss tears.
- Malignancy.

Q2 What are the surgical options if the bleeding is due to a bleeding peptic ulcer?

(Difficult Question)

- Under-running of the bleeding vessel.
- Excision of the ulcer.
- Gastrectomy.

Q3 What is the Rockall score?

(Honours Question)

■ This a prognostic scoring system for acute upper GI bleeds based on the patient's medical history, current clinical condition and endoscopic findings:

Table 8.1: Rockall score

Variable	Score
Age	0: <60 years 1: 60–80 years 2: >80 years
Shock	0: None 1: HR > 100; systolic blood pressure (SBP) > 100 2: HR > 100; SBP < 100
Comorbidity	0: None 2: Any major condition 3: Renal failure, liver failure, malignancy
Diagnosis	0: Mallory-Weiss Tear 1: All other causes except malignancy 2: Malignancy
Endoscopy	0: No bleeding visible 2: Visible blood or clot; spurting vessel

■ A score of >8: High risk of death.
■ A score of <3: Excellent prognosis.

Case 3: Acutely ischaemic leg

Instructions: This man, a known arteriopath, has presented with an acutely painful, pulseless leg. How would you manage him?

Key features to mention:

Viva discussion

■ **Recognise urgency.**
■ **Initial resuscitation:** *See above*, including IV fluids and opiate analgesia.
■ **Emergency investigations:** Angiogram in incomplete ischaemia; but do not delay definitive treatment if there is complete ischaemia.
■ **Additional monitoring:** CVP line and catheter to accurately guide resuscitation.
■ **Call for help:** Call early, as time is of the essence in this condition; if ischaemia is present for <6 hours, then it is still reversible.

- **Assess severity:** Document the six P's (*see below*).
- **Definitive treatment:** Depends on the cause.
  - In general, keep NBM preoperatively, and consider Heparinisation.
  - <u>Embolic cause:</u>
    - Embolectomy with a Fogarty catheter and on-table angiography.
    - Thrombolysis if embolectomy is unsuccessful.
    - Emergency reconstruction, with the possibility of a fasciotomy.
    - Amputation.
  - <u>Thrombotic cause:</u>
    - Thrombolysis with, e.g. streptokinase.
    - Angioplasty; stent insertion.
    - Emergency reconstruction or amputation if unsalvageable.

Completion

Viva questions

Q1 What are the signs of acute limb ischaemia?
- This is known as the six P's:
  - Pain: Usually severe.
  - Pallor: Occurs in progressive stages:
    - A white appearance progressing to mottled but blanching.
    - Next, non-blanching, mottled skin.
    - Finally, fixed staining and liquefaction.
  - Perishingly cold.
  - Pulseless: Confirm this with a doppler probe.
  - Paresthesiae: Assess sensation.
  - Paralysis: Assess motor function.
- Paresthesiae and paralysis are late signs, and by then the condition is usually irreversible.

Q2 What specific post-operative complication should you look for?

(Difficult Question)

- **Reperfusion injury,** which occurs when the limb's arterial oxygen supply is reintroduced; this leads to oxygen-free radicals, causing endothelial damage.
- This can lead to metabolic complications such as acidosis, ARDS and myoglobinaemia, or it can lead to a **compartment syndrome,** which requires an emergency fasciotomy.

Case 4: Ruptured abdominal aortic aneurysm

Instructions: This man was found collapsed in the street. He has a pulsatile, expansile mass on abdominal examination. How would you manage him?
- **Recognise urgency**
- **Initial resuscitation:** *See above*, including blood (do not wait for cross-matched blood; give O negative blood if available); maintain BP <90 mmHg, as you may destabilise a tamponading clot (permissive hypotension); no less than two large-bore cannulae, as you need to give fluids rapidly.

Authors' Top Tip

It takes up to an hour for cross-matched blood to be ready, and 30 minutes for type-specific blood. If your patient needs blood immediately, then use O negative blood. However, you must still CX, as the patient will require far more units intraoperatively.

- **Emergency investigations:** None required; go straight to theatre. Ensure you take bloods for CX (10 U).
- **Additional monitoring:** CVP line and urinary catheter.
- **Call for help:** Call for help as soon as you diagnose, as the patient needs immediate surgery.
- **Definitive treatment:**
  - Immediate surgery to cross-clamp the aorta proximal to the rupture and control the bleeding.
  - ITU care postoperatively.

Completion

Be cautious with the 60-year-old man who presents with renal colic; this may be a leaking AAA. And do not under any circumstances send an unstable patient for a CT abdomen; they will almost certainly arrest. One of our consultants used to call the CT scanner the 'donut of death' for this very reason.

Authors' Top Tip

If you must take a critically ill patient to the CT scanner, do not go alone – preferably take the anaesthetist with you!

Case 5: Post-operative fever

Instructions: This woman is 5 days post left hemicolectomy for a sigmoid cancer. The nurses have called you, as she has spiked a temperature. How would you manage her?

- **Recognise urgency.**
- **Initial resuscitation:** This involves a quick, systematic examination to look for a cause, i.e. listen to the chest for basal atelectasis, examine the abdomen for peritonitis, look at the wound for signs of infection and examine the legs for DVT. Assess for SIRS (*see* below).
- **Emergency investigations:** Do a septic screen, i.e. FBC, urine dipstick, CXR and culture any peripheral or central lines. Take blood cultures before you start antibiotics and a MC&S of any drain fluid. Consider a water-soluble contrast study of the rectum to rule out an anastomotic leak.
- **Call for help:** The patient may require surgery for a possible anastomotic leak.
- **Definitive treatment:** Depends on the cause:
  - Keep patient NBM, if not already.
  - **Urine or chest infection:** Give empirical IV antibiotics as per local protocol and chest physiotherapy for basal atelectasis. If the patient is in septic shock, then give a fluid challenge and consider increasing the level of care to HDU.
  - **Anastomotic leak:** If the patient is stable and the leak is small, then conservative management is preferred. If peritonitic, consider laparotomy for a wash out and to plug the leak.

Completion

The most common cause of postoperative fever in abdominal surgery is basal atelectasis. This can be prevented with good chest physiotherapy and adequate analgesia. Some patients undergoing major abdominal surgery are on epidural analgesia for this very reason. Being able to take good, painless deep breaths and clear secretions is essential in preventing this life-threatening complication. Anastomotic leaks typically occur between days 3 and 5 but can occur at any time. Always bear this in mind.

Viva questions

Q1 What are the causes of postoperative fever?

Table 8.2: Postoperative fever

Post-op period	Aetiology
Immediate	**<24 hours:** Physiological stress response to surgery
Early	**<3 days:** Basal atelectasis (pneumonia) **>3 days:** Pneumonia, wound infection, anastomotic leaks, subphrenic or pelvic abscess, UTI, line infection (central and peripheral) **>5 days:** PE or DVT

The time periods are only a guide, so always examine the patient and investigate as appropriate.

Q2   What is SIRS?

(Difficult Question)

- This stands for systemic inflammatory response syndrome and has at least two of the following features:
    - **Temperature:** >38°C or <36° C.
    - **Pulse:** >90/minute.
    - **Respiratory rate:** >20/minute.
    - **White cell count:** >12 or <4.

There is a spectrum of disorders in sepsis, ranging from SIRS to severe sepsis, where there is evidence of one or more organ dysfunction in a patient with a confirmed site of infection. Do not underestimate sepsis, especially in an elderly patient. There is a Surviving Sepsis campaign being implemented throughout NHS trusts. Being aware of the sepsis care bundles would certainly impress the examiner.

Case 6: Postoperative oliguria

Instructions: This woman has returned to the ward after having had a laparotomy for acute abdominal pain. The nurses ring you, as her hourly urine output has been <30 mL. How would you manage her?

- **Recognise urgency.**
- **Initial resuscitation:** This involves a quick, systematic examination to assess volume status:
    - **Mental status:** Confusion is a sign of cerebral hypoperfusion.
    - **Hands:** Check for decreased skin turgor, a prolonged capillary refill time and whether the patient is cool and clammy.
    - **Vital signs:** Note the presence of tachycardia and/or hypotension.
    - **Assess jugular venous pressure (JVP):** A low JVP suggests hypovolaemia and is best demonstrated when the patient is lying supine, as JVP is normally visible in this position. If the patient is on a CVP line, check if there is a low reading *(see below)*.
    - **Examine:** Look at the chest for signs of fluid overload; check the abdomen for a distended bladder, as seen in obstruction.
    - **Fluid balance chart assessment:**
        - **Pattern:** Is the oliguria abrupt or gradual? Complete anuria when previously there was adequate urine flow suggests acute catheter blockage.
        - **Excessive fluid loss:** Look at the fluid output, especially the drains, fistulae or stomas; are there any excessive fluid losses that have not been compensated for?
        - **Inadequate fluid intake:** What is the daily fluid input, and is there enough fluid being given to the patient to balance output? Remember, some operations can result in significant fluid loss, which needs to be replaced. Aim for a slightly positive fluid balance.

> ### Authors' Top Tip
>
> *Whenever you assess a post-operative patient with oliguria, always read the operative notes, as this scenario may have been anticipated by the operating surgeon. In fact, the surgeon may have left specific postoperative instructions on how to manage this.*

- **Emergency investigations:** Check renal function; the urea and creatinine may be markedly raised due to dehydration or renal failure, and always compare these to previous readings to assess whether this rise is acute or chronic. Hypovolaemia due to blood loss leads to a reduced renal perfusion pressure and causes pre-renal failure. A raised Hb or haematocrit is also an indicator of dehydration. Consider giving the patient a fluid challenge, which can also be a therapeutic measure *(see below)*.
- **Additional monitoring:** The patient may need CVP monitoring if she is not responding to fluid challenges. A urinary catheter is essential to accurately monitor urine output, and in cases of post-renal obstruction causing oliguria, this is the initial treatment. Keep a strict fluid balance chart to monitor response to treatment.
- **Call for help:** Patients may require surgery for possible intra-abdominal bleeding, as a cause for hypovolaemia in for example a post nephrectomy patient. And some may require HDU care for CVP line monitoring.
- **Definitive treatment:** This depends on the cause:
  - **Post-renal:** Usually due to obstruction by a large stone or BPH causing acute urinary retention. Insert a urinary catheter, or check that a pre-existing one is not blocked.
  - **Intrinsic renal:** Call for expert help. The patient may need dialysis in the interim period.
  - **Pre-renal:** Give a fluid challenge and reassess:
    - ❏ The basic principle of a fluid challenge is to give a small amount of fluid quickly and assess the response.
    - ❏ Whichever fluid you use is a matter of personal preference; some use normal saline or Hartmann's solution. We suggest using a colloid, as this stays in the intravascular compartment longer and can unmask haemorrhage as a cause of hypovolaemia.
    - ❏ Give 250 mL of Gelofusine as a stat bolus intravenously, then assess the patient's response by examining her volume status (as described above), looking particularly at the vital signs and urine output for signs of improvement, i.e. the tachycardia and BP should start to normalise, and the urine output will pick up towards normal.

> ### Authors' Top Tip
>
> *Pre-renal failure is the most common cause of postoperative oliguria and is most likely due to hypovolaemia secondary to dehydration.*

❏   If the patient is unresponsive to the initial fluid challenge, then repeat the challenge and reassess the patient.
❏   If there is still no response or an inadequate response, then consider a CVP line to accurately assess fluid volume status (usually you would need a senior review at this point to sanction the CVP line).
❏   CVP line monitoring: CVP normal values are 3–7 cm/H2O; although remember it is the pattern of response to a fluid challenge rather than absolute numbers that are informative.

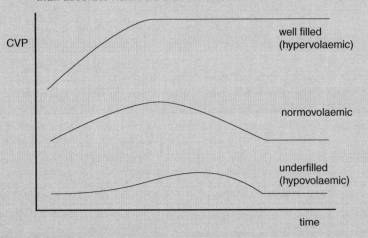

Figure 8.1: CVP monitoring

–   **Patient is underfilled:** CVP will rise in response to a challenge, then fall back down to the original value quickly.
–   **Patient is normovolaemic:** CVP will rise substantially and will fall back down, but over a longer period of time.
–   **Patient is well filled:** CVP will rise substantially, but will not fall.
   ❏   If the patient is unresponsive despite several fluid challenges, consider blood loss as a possible cause and call your senior for urgent review after having thoroughly examined the patient for potential sites of blood loss. The patient may require a blood transfusion whilst awaiting an urgent laparotomy to find the source of bleeding if one cannot be identified on the ward.
   ❏   If the patient is underfilled as a result of excessive fluid losses and is not responsive to fluid challenges on the ward, then she may need a higher level of care, e.g. HDU for monitoring.

Completion

Always read the operative notes to see if there were any unexpected complications or specific advice with regards to fluid management. Hypovolaemia could simply be due to dehydration but could also be as a result of ongoing haemorrhage, illustrating the importance of a focused clinical examination. Normal urine output is 0.5 mL/kg/hour, which equates to roughly 30–35 mL/hour in a 70 kg man.

8.2 THE TRAUMA CALL

Advanced Trauma Life Support (ATLS) is a standardised method for simultaneously assessing and treating a multiply injured patient. The initial assessment is essentially the same as for any emergency, but with an emphasis on Airway with **cervical spine immobilisation** and Circulation with **haemorrhage control**.

Although in actual clinical practise there is often a dedicated trauma team, you should consider yourself to be alone for purposes of the viva.

Case 1: Trauma call

Instructions: This man was involved in an RTA. There are no obvious sites of injury. The ambulance crew stated he is persistently hypotensive despite adequate resuscitation in the field. His GCS is <8. How would you manage him?

- **Recognise urgency:** State that you would manage the patient according to ATLS principles.
- **Initial resuscitation:** Request intubation; as the patient's GCS is less than eight, he cannot maintain his own airway and requires a definitive airway in the form of an endotracheal tube. You need expert help for this; the anaesthetist will need to be quickly paged. Use no less than two large-bore cannulae. Specifically, consider causes of hypotension in your primary survey and look for a cause. As above, begin with 2 L of Hartmann's solution, and if no response, give blood. If the patient is unstable, do not wait for cross-matched blood, you can give O negative blood if available.
- **Emergency investigations:** CXR, pelvic X-ray, C-spine. FAST scan to look for a source of bleeding. CT head/chest/abdo/pelvis if stable.
- **Additional monitoring:** A urinary catheter should be inserted once you have excluded a high-riding prostate on PR exam, and there are no obvious signs of urethral damage, as indicated by the presence of blood at the meatus or perineal bruising.
- **Call for help:** Call for help early; often there is a dedicated trauma team.
- **Definitive treatment:** As this patient is persistently hypotensive, this suggests blood loss:
  - You must **identify the source of bleeding** by looking in the following five places: the abdomen, the chest, the long bones/pelvis, the head and the floor.
  - **Treat the underlying cause:** Intra-abdominal bleeding will require immediate laparotomy to identify the source and control the haemorrhage. In this case, there is no need for further investigation.

Completion

Depending on the clinical scenario your examiner takes, you could offer treatment options for any of the five common sources of bleeding; if the patient had a haemothorax in the chest, you could describe how to insert a chest drain (*see* Chapter 11, Surgical procedures: Case 3); if the source is the head, then you could discuss management of raised intracranial pressure (*see* Chapter 12, Case 3: Viva Q4).

Viva questions

Q1 How do you assess hypovolaemic shock?

(Difficult Question)

- Through clinical examination and assessment:

Table 8.3: Stages of hypovolaemia

Variable	Class I	Class II	Class III	Class IV
Blood loss (%)	0–15	15–30	30–40	>40
Blood loss (volume)	750 mL	750 mL–1.5 L	1.5 L to 2 L	>2 L
Mental status	Alert/slightly anxious	Anxious	Aggressive, confused	Lethargic, unconscious
Pulse	<100	>100	>120	>140
Blood pressure	Normal	Normal	Decreased	Un-recordable
Urine output (mL/hour)	>30	20–30	5–15	Nil

Authors' Top Tip

Do not overly rely on a stable BP, as patients need to be in stage III shock for there to be a discernable drop in BP. Remember, patients can deteriorate rapidly!

Q2 What is a FAST scan?

(Honours Question)

- This stands for focussed assessment sonogram in trauma (*see* www.trauma.org/archive/radiology/FASTfast.html).
- This is a rapid, bedside ultrasound examination of various parts of the body where blood is likely to have collected post-trauma. This includes looking at the:
  - **Abdomen:** The perihepatic, perisplenic and pelvic spaces.
  - **Thorax:** At the pericardium.
- Although usually used to look for blood loss, it is now seen as an extension of the clinical examination and with expert hands this can be performed in less than a minute to look for various pathologies.

CHAPTER 9

Vascular

Vascular pathology is an important part of surgical clinical finals. You will no doubt see a vascular case of some sort in finals. It is therefore imperative that you are familiar with the arterial supply of both the upper and lower limbs and are confident in taking a vascular-orientated history to illicit the salient points that will confirm a diagnosis of vascular disease (*see* Chapter 2, Case 3).

Peripheral vascular disease is also known as peripheral arterial disease (PAD), or vascular occlusive disease, and can be either acute or chronic. It results from obstruction of the large arteries in the peripheries, i.e. the arms or the legs. Obstruction can arise as a result of atherosclerosis, thromboembolic disease or inflammatory stenosis, which results in ischaemia of the peripheries.

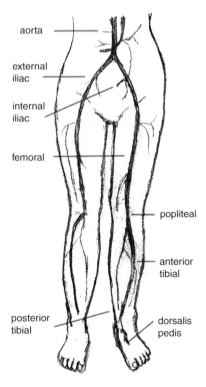

aorta

external
iliac

internal
iliac

femoral

popliteal

anterior
tibial

posterior
tibial

dorsalis
pedis

Figure 9.1: Arterial supply of lower limbs

9.1 PERIPHERAL VASCULAR EXAMINATION

The vascular examination is aimed at eliciting signs of vascular disease and should be part of the cardiovascular examination in general, but for the purposes of the examination you will most likely be asked to concentrate your efforts on one aspect of this, e.g. the lower limb peripheral vascular system. When asked to perform an examination of the peripheral vascular system, it is often safest to begin with the hands and examine the upper and lower limb vasculature in a standard format. However, examiners may direct you to the lower limbs to save time. Below, we describe a complete peripheral vascular examination that can be adapted to the situation you find yourself in; you may find that you need to omit various sections to adapt to the scenario posed.

Authors' Top Tip

Remember, the majority of features in peripheral vascular disease are found in the observation section of the examination, so say what you see and you will improve your chances of scoring highly.

Clinical examination

Introduction
As for any clinical encounter (*see* Chapter 1, Principles of a clinical encounter).

General inspection
✔ **Paraphernalia of disease**
- Does the patient have an amputation? If so, describe the level (*see* Viva Q5). Are there any associated walking/mobility aids or prosthesis?
- The patient may be on oxygen, an IV infusion of heparin may be running, there may be GTN spray and/or cigarettes may be clearly visible by the bedside.

Upper limb vascular examination
✔ **Examine the hands**
- **Skin changes:** Look for tar staining, tendon palmar xanthoma (seen in hypercholesterolaemia), and purple discolouration of the fingertips (atheroembolism).
- **Muscle wasting:** Wasting of the small muscles of the hand (thoracic outlet syndrome).
- **Temperature:** Palpate the hands for temperature, which may be cold in PAD.
- **Pulses:** Assess the radial and brachial pulses on both arms; comment on rate, rhythm and character.
- **Capillary refill time:** Measure the capillary refill time (in a normal person, this should be less than 2 seconds).
- **Blood pressure:** Record the blood pressure at the arm, then compare the blood pressure of both arms; there should be no more than a 15 mmHg difference between the two sides in the absence of arterial disease.

✔ **Examine the neck and face**
  ▪ **Eyes:** Look for corneal arcus, xanthelasma (signs of hypercholesterolaemia) and conjunctival pallor (anaemia).
  ▪ **Mouth:** Look for central cyanosis (bluish tinge to lips and buccal mucosa) and angular stomatitis (anaemia).
  ▪ **Neck:** Inspect for prominent veins on the neck, anterior chest wall and over the shoulders; the presence of these indicates axillary or subclavian vein occlusion.
  ▪ **Pulses:** Feel for the carotid pulse; remember, one side at a time! This is best felt with the patient's head resting on a pillow in the supine position and the patient looking in the opposite direction to you; feel under the sternocleidomastoid muscle with the tips of your index and middle fingers.
  ▪ **Bruits:** Auscultate for carotid bruits using the bell of your stethoscope.

Abdominal examination
✔ **Examine for arterial disease in the abdomen**
  ▪ The abdominal examination typically involves actively ruling out an abdominal aortic aneurysm.
  ▪ For more details (*see* Case 1).

Lower limb vascular examination
✔ **General inspection**
  ▪ **Asymmetry:** Look for any obvious lower limb asymmetry.
    – **Amputation:** Has there been an amputation? If so, describe the level of the amputation and mention if this is confined to one lower limb or both limbs.
    – **Oedema:** If present, is it localised around one area, or is it generalised? Note the level and if would you describe this to be pitting oedema.
    – **Muscle wasting:** Mention if this is bilateral/unilateral/symmetrical.
  ▪ **Surgical scars:** Are these indicative of previous varicose vein removal, or are the scars suggestive of vein harvesting for a CABG? Note any obvious varicosities present.
  ▪ **Skin changes:**
    – **Discolouration:** Erythema, pallor, brown (haemosiderin deposits), purple or black from haemostasis.
    – **Venous guttering:** In the presence of severe ischaemia, the veins collapse and appear like gutters in the subcutaneous tissue.
    – **Trophic changes:** Such as absence of hair, shiny skin, gangrene.
    – **Ulcers:** If seen, describe as you would an ulcer (*see* Examination of ulcers).
✔ **Closer inspection**
  ▪ Detailed inspection of the toes:
    – Look for any toe amputations.
    – Look for purple discolouration of the toes/forefoot (due to atheroembolism from an AAA – the so-called 'trash foot').
    – Look carefully at the tips of the toes and between all the toes for areas of gangrene or ulcers (this involves actually separating the toes with your hands and looking carefully!).

- Focus on pressure areas where ischaemic ulcers can develop, specifically:
  - The lateral malleolus and lateral aspect of the foot.
  - The sole of the foot for ulceration of the metatarsal heads.
  - The heels, where neuropathic ulcers may be found (this involves lifting the patient's foot to get a view of the heel, so ask the patient if he or she has any pain before you do this).
- Examine any ulcers found (*see* Section 9.3: Cases 1, 2).

Palpation

✔ **Check skin temperature**
  - This is a marker of perfusion (blood flow in the dermal vessels).
  - Using the back of your hands, compare the temperature of both legs, first starting most distally then working your way up to become more proximal.
  - Cool legs/feet suggest peripheral vascular disease.
✔ **Check capillary refill time**
  - This is performed by pressing down with your fingers on the pulp of the big toe for 5 seconds, then releasing; the toes should blanch and return to their normal colour in less than 2 seconds. Compare both sides.
  - If the toes take longer than this to return to their normal colour, inform the examiner you would like to perform Buerger's test.
  - It is important to remember that a prolonged capillary refill time may be falsely elevated if the patient is generally cold or shut down peripherally.
✔ **Perform Buerger's test**
  - This test involves straight-leg raising with the patient in a supine position. Before attempting to perform this test, ask the patient if he or she has any pain in the knees or hips.
  - Begin by elevating both legs to 45°, holding on to the legs just proximal to the ankles for a minimum of 1 minute.

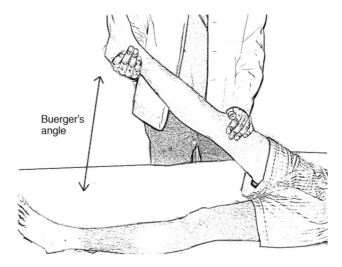

Figure 9.2: Buerger's angle

- During this time, in an individual with PAD you will see venous guttering as the superficial veins empty, and the legs will turn pale as the blood drains away.
- After this time period, reassess the soles of the patient's feet. If the soles have turned white, this is a strong indication of ischaemia. Remember to compare both sides, as this is often more important than the changes seen in one foot alone.
- Then ask the patient to sit up and lower his or her legs and feet off the couch. Watch how long it takes the veins in the legs to refill; note the colour change in the legs and feet.

Authors' Top Tip

In actual clinical practise you may need to give the patient a hand to help the patient sit up.

- In someone unaffected by peripheral arterial disease, the legs should turn pink, but in someone with PAD you will see them turning to a bluish colour from the deoxygenated blood as it travels over the ischaemic tissues and then turns red from the reactive hyperaemia from post-hypoxic vasodilation. This can take up to 2 minutes in someone with poor peripheral circulation. If this occurs, the test is considered to be positive and indicates severe PAD.

This test is now considered to be outdated and can often be omitted; only perform the test if the examiner asks you to do so when you offer.

Traditionally, there were two parts to Buerger's test: first, checking the angle at which the leg goes pale (Beurger's angle), then the time taken for the legs to reperfuse. In theory, the legs in a normal patient should remain pink and well perfused up to an angle of more than 90°. In actual practise, lifting a patient's leg by flexing the hip to 90° whilst keeping the knee fully extended can be difficult to achieve, especially in patients who have multiple co-morbidities. We suggest you omit this part and check for the perfusion time rather than being concerned with angles.

There is a difference of opinion when classifying severe ischaemia and critical ischaemia in terms of Beurger's angle. If asked this in a viva situation, mention that there is some discrepancy in its exact definition but that a Buerger's angle of <50° suggests severe ischaemia, while an angle of <20–25° suggests critical ischaemia.

Peripheral pulses

Before the examination, make sure you are efficient at feeling for pulses, as they are not always easy to find, especially the foot pulses.

Authors' Top Tip

The key to accurately feeling for pedal pulses is to know your anatomy and thereby the location of the pulse and to press lightly, not deeply (as this accentuates your own pulse), and to practise as often as possible.

The popliteal pulse is notoriously difficult to palpate, and if in the examination you feel the popliteal pulse very easily, this is probably an aneurysm and not a reflection of your examination skills!

Classically, you work proximally to distally, palpating each artery systematically, comparing the strength on both sides and recording your findings as: present, reduced, absent or aneurysmal. It is equally acceptable to palpate distal to proximal, so long as you are systematic in your approach. Some candidates prefer to auscultate after palpating each individual artery; this is also acceptable but time-consuming. We suggest you to focus your auscultation to specific arteries, as advised below.

✔ **Palpate for the femoral pulse**
  ■ The femoral artery is anatomically located at the mid-inguinal point, which is a point halfway between the anterior superior iliac spine (ASIS) and the pubic tubercle.
  ■ It is found in the femoral triangle between the femoral nerve and femoral vein; remember the mnemonic Nerve Artery Vein Y-fronts (NAVY: lateral to medial).

Authors' Top Tip

Remember to tell the patient what you are doing before you palpate the femoral artery. You are invading the patient's personal space by palpating his groin!

✔ **Palpate for the popliteal pulse**
  ■ The popliteal artery is located at the lower margin of the popliteal fossa between the two heads of the gastrocnemius muscle.
  ■ Flex the knee to >10° and place the thumbs of both hands on the anterior aspect of the knee, then gently palpate in an upwards direction in the popliteal fossa with your index and middle fingers.
  ■ Many people find this to be a very difficult pulse to palpate; often the pulse is lower than you think, so practice before the examination.
  ■ If the pulse is extremely easy to palpate, consider the possibility of a popliteal aneurysm, as this is the second-most common site after the abdomen for the development of an aneurysm.

✔ **Palpate for the posterior tibial pulse**
  ■ This is found just posterior and 2 cm inferior to the medial malleolus of the tibia.

✔ **Palpate for the dorsalis pedis pulse**
  ■ This is sometimes difficult to find, even in normal people, and is absent or abnormally sited in 10% of individuals.
  ■ It is found on the dorsal aspect of the foot, just lateral to the extensor hallucis longus tendon.
  ■ Ask the patient to dorsiflex his great toe, which will accentuate the tendon to the naked eye, then palpate immediately lateral to this and move proximally slowly along the tendon to locate the pulse.

Auscultation
✔ **Listen for bruits over the femoral artery**
  ■ Listen at the femoral artery and in the adductor canal for the superficial femorals.

✔ **Listen for bruits in the abdomen over the aorta and iliac vessels**
- You may also hear bruits over the renal artery.

If you have not already done so in the upper limb vascular examination, check the carotid arteries for bruits. Remember that bruits suggest stenosis of the vessels.

Special tests
✔ **Measure ankle brachial pressure index (ABPI) on both sides**
- ABPI is a non-invasive method of determining the presence and severity of peripheral vascular disease. This method calls for a hand-held doppler probe and a sphygmomanometer.
- It examines for a fall in blood pressure in the arteries supplying the legs, which occurs as a result of occlusive arterial disease in the arteries supplying the lower limbs.
- The index is calculated by taking the higher of the two systolic blood pressures at the ankle (over the posterior tibial pulse) or at the foot (the dorsalis pedis pulse) and dividing by the systolic blood pressure at the brachial artery in the arm:

$$ABPI_{Leg} = \frac{P_{Leg}}{P_{Arm}}$$

- **Method of carrying out the ABPI:**
  - A sphygmomanometer cuff is inflated just proximal to the ankle joint, whilst a doppler probe is placed over the posterior tibial pulse and the cuff is inflated until the noise from the doppler signal disappears.
  - The cuff is then slowly deflated until the signal in the doppler reappears. This is taken as the systolic pressure reading at the foot.
  - This can then be repeated with the doppler probe over the dorsalis pedis pulse; the higher of the two readings is generally used in the equation to work out the ABPI. The higher of the two systolic readings from the arms is used.
- **Interpretation of results:**
  - A value of >0.9 is considered normal, <0.8 claudication, <0.3 critical ischaemia.
  - You can get false positive results, e.g. an ABPI of >1.2 suggests hardening of the arteries from calcification, resulting in the arteries being stiffer or less compressible. This is seen in patients with diabetes mellitus and in renal failure.
  - Sometimes ABPI is used as part of the 'walk test', where patients are walked on a treadmill to measure their maximal claudication distance. The ABPI is measured before and after; a drop of >20% suggests significant arterial disease.

Complete the examination
✔ **Further examination**
- *'To complete my examination, I would like to perform a complete lower limb orthopaedic examination and a neurological examination, looking particularly at motor power and sensation'.*

If you were asked to skip the abdominal or upper limb examination, then make sure you mention that you would check for an AAA and examine the rest of the peripheral vascular system. If you haven't done Buerger's test already, then offer to do so now. A musculoskeletal and neurological examination is required, as occlusive arterial disease can affect both systems, and in addition, features such as paralysis and paraesthesiae are features of critical ischaemia.

✔ **Thank the patient**
✔ **Wash your hands**
✔ **Present your findings**

Viva questions

Q1 How would you investigate this patient?
   ■ The patient will require imaging in the form of a duplex scan and an angiogram to assess the degree of stenosis and the presence of any distal runoff.

(Good Response)

'Investigations can be divided into bedside tests, blood tests and imaging':

Simple bedside tests I would like to perform include:
   ■ *Checking the patient's BM, as he or she is likely to be diabetic.*
   ■ *An ECG for evidence of coexisting heart disease, as the patient is likely to be an arteriopath.*

Simple blood tests I would like to perform include:
   ■ *FBC to check for anaemia or polycythaemia.*
   ■ *U&Es to check the patient's renal function, which is particularly important if undergoing contrast studies, especially in diabetics (contrast-induced nephropathy).*
   ■ *Serum lipid profile for hypercholesterolaemia to address risk factor modification.*
   ■ *Clotting for the presence of a coagulopathy or for monitoring purposes in patients on anticoagulants (APTT for those on heparin infusions who presented acutely with critical ischaemia).*
   ■ *G&S in case the patient undergoes operative management.*
   ■ *ESR to screen for vasculitides and a specialist antinuclear autoantibodies (ANA) screen for selected patients.*

Imaging I would like to request will include:
   ■ *'CXR to look for coexisting cardio respiratory disease, particularly as part of a preoperative assessment.*
   ■ *I would also request specialist imaging to assess the extent of disease and help plan operative management:*
      – *Specifically, a duplex scan to check for the degree of stenosis.*
      – *A spiral CT to reconstruct 3D images of vessels noninvasively.*

> – *And in some patients, a digital subtraction angiogram (DSA) to demonstrate the level of blockage, runoff and the presence of a collateral blood supply'.*

(Honours Response)

Those who undergo invasive imaging such as angiography have a catheter introduced (using the Seldinger technique) into the femoral artery and guided to the site of the lesion, where radio-dense contrast is injected and imaged using X-rays; the stenosis can be treated at the same time by balloon angioplasty. A DSA uses computer software to subtract bones and soft tissues from the image so that the arterial supply is demonstrated in high resolution, with the consequent advantage of using less contrast material.

Q2 Can you estimate the extent of stenosis from a hand-held doppler probe?

(Difficult Question)

- A simple, hand-held doppler probe detects arterial pulsation as an audible signal.
- The degree of stenosis causes turbulent blood flow, which results in bruits heard on auscultation with a stethoscope.
- Characteristic waveforms are seen when using a doppler probe:
  - **Normal vessels:** Triphasic waveform.
  - **Mild stenosis:** Biphasic waveform.
  - *Severe* **stenosis:** Monophasic waveform.

In the outpatient setting, this can be a useful screening test. If you have never tried it, practise on yourself and listen to the pulsation of your radial artery; the probe uses the principles of the Doppler effect to convert the movement of blood in your artery to a signal, which is displayed as an audible noise. If you listen carefully, you will hear a triple waveform, which will confirm normal flow. Students often say that they expect to hear a double noise coinciding with their pulse, but this shows a lack of experience with the hand-held probe.

   You will not be expected to have a great understanding of the probe, but certainly knowing the above will stand you in good stead with the examiner should he ask; or, as we suggest, you should offer to the examiner whilst you are locating the pulse for an ABPI measurement. There is no harm in saying you can hear a triphasic waveform, suggesting good flow in that vessel.

Examiner's Anecdote

'When he told me he could hear the normal triphasic waveform at the posterior tibial artery, I felt like shaking his hand. I was very impressed indeed!'

Q3 Why are the lower limbs more commonly affected by PAD when compared to the upper limbs?
- The arterial supply to the legs is not as well developed as the arterial supply to the upper limbs.

- Consequently, the lower limb arterial supply is also more susceptible to atherosclerosis than the upper limbs; as a result, PAD is approximately eight times more common in the lower limbs than in the upper limbs.

Q4 How would you treat this patient with lower limb occlusive arterial disease?

This involves a MDT management approach. In general, however, management can be divided into conservative, medical or surgical measures. Conservative and medical measures focus around the modification of risk factors.

Conservative measures include:
- Stopping smoking.
- Change in diet as part of the treatment of obesity.
- Early liaison with a diabetic specialist nurse to achieve good diabetic control.
- Referral to a podiatrist for foot care.
- A dedicated exercise program (in those with intermittent claudication) to encourage collateral supply build-up.

Medical measures include:
- Aspirin (75 mg) for life, unless contraindicated.
- Treatment of hypertension.
- Treatment of high cholesterol with statins.
- Treatment of diabetes.

Surgical procedures include:
- Endovascular techniques with stents and grafting.
- Reconstructive surgery resulting in a bypass of the occlusion; this can be anatomical (fem-pop bypass) or extra-anatomical (axillo-femoral bypass).
- Amputation (when the limb is not salvageable).

Other operative measures such as endarterectomy, where the atheromatous plaque is cored out, is commonly used in surgery for carotid artery stenosis. Sympathectomies can be beneficial in those with chronic, intractable pain.

(Good Response)

Authors' Top Tip

Remember that this is a chronic condition, so ensure you mention the role of the MDT somewhere in your answer!

Q5 What are the benefits of a below-knee amputation (BKA) over an above-knee amputation (AKA)?

(Honours Question)

- BKAs are preferred, as:
  - Patients typically demonstrate better mobility and are less likely to be wheelchair bound, thereby increasing their chances of successful rehabilitation and a better quality of life.
  - The physical benefits include preserving the limb length and reducing the energy required to mobilise, as compared to the complications of an AKA.
  - Studies have shown that life expectancy for those with an AKA is poor when compared to those with a BKA.
  - Furthermore, patients with an AKA are more likely to develop critical ischaemia in the other leg.

Although you may not be expected to recognise the different types of amputations or to be able to examine one competently at an undergraduate level, you should at the very least be able to differentiate between an AKA and a BKA, which is usually self-evident.

Also, be sure you know some of the reasons for amputation; the so-called 'three D's': Dead Limb (vascular, e.g. peripheral vascular disease); Dangerous Limb (infection, e.g. oestomyelitis) and Debilitating Limb (trauma, e.g. frostbite).

Case 1: Abdominal aortic aneurysm

Instructions: Please examine this man's abdomen as part of your vascular examination.

Key features to look for:

Inspection

- There may be abdominal scars, particularly over the femorals, from previous bypass surgery.
- There may be an obvious mass in the epigastrium, or visible pulsations (sometimes these are easier to see from the side of the bed by kneeling down to the height of the patient and looking across, e.g. *'I can see visible pulsations in the upper abdominal wall'*).

Palpation/auscultation

- Gently palpate above and slightly to the left of the umbilicus (before the aorta bifurcates at the L4 level) using the tips of the fingers on both hands, palpating progressively deeper if necessary (stop if this causes the patient pain).
- This will demonstrate pulsatility as your hands move with each pulse, but you need to palpate for a pulsatile and expansile mass. Remember, a pulsatile mass could just occur as a result of transmitted pulsations, so you need to establish whether this is also expansile.
- To demonstrate expansibility, place one hand on either side of the mass, and you should see your hands moving laterally with each pulse.

- Now estimate the transverse diameter of the mass in centimetres.
- Try to feel the upper border of the mass, which if felt would suggest the aneurysm is infrarenal (only 1% are suprarenal).
- Auscultate the aneurysm for bruits.
- Specifically examine the femoral and popliteal pulse to confirm it is present and in case these arteries are also aneurysmal (AAA increases incidence of other aneurysms).

Completion
Usually this case is seen as part of the peripheral vascular examination but can and has come up before in finals as a separate case. If the instructions are to perform an abdominal examination, then examine as you would an abdomen, e.g. by starting at the hands. If you are asked to examine the peripheral vascular system, then stick to your routine. Some examiners may rush you along to examine the abdomen and make you skip sections. Do not be flustered; they are often trying to save time and really just want to viva you!

Viva questions

Q1 What is an aneurysm?
- A pathological, localised, permanent dilatation of an artery to more than 1.5 times its original diameter involving all three layers of its parent wall.

(Surgical Definition)

Authors' Top Tip

Remember, a pseudoaneurysm doesn't involve all three layers of the arterial wall. Examiners love their definitions, so know this definition cold!

Q2 What are the potential complications of an AAA?
- Rupture, dissection, thrombosis and embolisation from the thrombosis, leading to trash foot.
- Fistula formation into adjacent organs, such as the colon (especially the duodenum), or the vena cava.

A fistula is an abnormal connection between two epithelial surfaces lined by granulation tissue.

(Surgical Definition)

Q3 What factors would make you consider elective operative treatment of an aneurysm?

(Difficult Question)

- This depends on two main features: if the patient is symptomatic or not.
- In patients who are asymptomatic, the United Kingdom Small Aneurysm Trial recommends repair when the aneurysm diameter is ≥5.5 cm, or if it is expanding at a rate of >1 cm a year.
- Symptomatic patients should have their aneurysm repaired.

Although a detailed understanding of operative treatment is not required at this stage in your career, for the more ambitious student it will stimulate an interesting viva discussion if you are aware of some of the current treatment options apart from open repair. Endovascular repair, which can be done by an interventional radiologist, is gaining popularity, as is laparoscopic repair in certain surgical centres. When we sat finals, the topical issue of screening patients for AAA was a possible direction to take the viva. Now that the NHS has begun a national programme, you may still be questioned with regards to whether it is a good screening program or not. If you do discuss screening, be aware of the current issues, and as a good starting point mention that such a program should ideally meet the Modified Wilson's criteria for screening programmes. This then allows you to demonstrate your understanding of epidemiology and helps structure your argument.

9.2 EXAMINATION OF VARICOSE VEINS

During finals, this is commonly seen in the vascular examination station, as there are plenty of subjects for the examiners to recruit.

The venous drainage of the lower limbs consists of the superficial and deep venous systems. The superficial system consists of the long and short saphenous veins and is responsible for draining the skin and subcutaneous tissues of the leg. The deep venous system exists within the muscles of the leg and is covered by fascia; it receives blood from the superficial venous system through the connecting perforating veins. When the muscles contract, blood is pushed towards the heart, and the valves in the veins are responsible for preventing backflow of blood. In cases where the valves have become incompetent, blood is forced from the deep system to the superficial system, causing the veins to dilate.

Varicose veins are dilated, tortuous and prominent veins of the superficial venous system of the lower limb seen in the distribution of the short and long saphenous veins.

(Surgical Definition)

There are a number of risk factors for the development of varicose veins, which include a history of DVT/PE, increasing age, obesity, a positive family history, pregnancy and pelvic masses (the latter two risk factors cause varicose veins by increasing pressure on the IVC and iliac veins). You should try to illicit the presence of these risk factors whilst taking a history.

Other points to remember include asking the patient about aching legs and swellings in the legs, whether the legs feel heavy, pruritus, restless legs and skin changes (venous eczema, ulcers). The patient will probably report that the symptoms become worse by the end of the day, especially in occupations that involve prolonged periods of standing.

Also enquire as to whether the patient has had any previous treatment to the leg or whether concern over the varicose veins is purely cosmetic. In a female patient, always enquire whether she is on the OCP, as this will need to be stopped at least 4 weeks before any surgical intervention due to the associated risks of DVT.

Do not feel daunted when presented with this case in the examination; proceed in a logical manner and stay calm.

Authors' Top Tip

Some students have in the past made the mistake of examining the patient supine and have missed varicosities altogether, only to be embarrassed by an examiner who asks the patient to stand up, with the varicosities becoming apparent. Therefore, always remember to inspect the patient lying down and standing up.

Clinical examination

Introduction
As for any clinical encounter (*see* Chapter 1, Principles of a clinical encounter). Specifically for this case:
✔ **Position patient appropriately:** The examination is performed with the patient in a supine position initially, and then the patient is required to stand up.

Inspection
✔ **Observe patient lying supine**
  ■ On general inspection, look for obvious lower-limb asymmetry, scars from previous varicose vein removal or vein harvesting for a CABG; note any obvious varicosities.
  ■ Look for signs of chronic venous insufficiency:
    – Lower-limb swelling and brown discolouration (hemosiderin deposition).
    – Telangiectasia and venous eczema.
    – Lipodermatosclerosis from chronic venous hypertension causing sclerosis of skin and subcutaneous tissues from fibrin deposition.
    – Erythema seen in thrombophlebitis.
  ■ Look specifically in the 'gaiter area' around the medial malleolus.
    – This is where venous ulcers are typically seen.
  ■ Look at the groin for hernias, a saphena varix or a prominent lymph node.
✔ **Observe patient standing**
  ■ Look for tortuous varicosities:
    – Anteriorly in the distribution of the great saphenous vein.
    – Posteriorly in the short saphenous vein distribution.

'Posteriorly I can see that there are multiple dilated and elongated veins in the distribution of the short saphenous vein'.

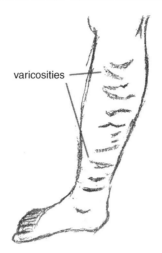

varicosities

Figure 9.3: Varicose veins

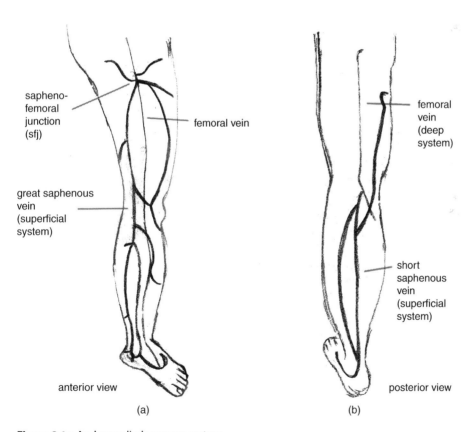

sapheno-
femoral
junction
(sfj)

femoral vein

great saphenous
vein
(superficial
system)

femoral
vein
(deep
system)

short
saphenous
vein
(superficial
system)

anterior view

posterior view

(a)

(b)

Figure 9.4a, b: Lower limb venous system

Remember that varicosities can also arise from calf perforators, and in some people the accessory vein of Giacomini, found on the posterior aspect of the thigh, may also become varicosed. It may be difficult to distinguish between great and short saphenous vein varicosities, especially below the knee.

Note that the patient remains standing until the tourniquet test.

Palpation

✔ **Palpate for a saphena varix**
- Locate the SFJ: it is found 2 cm inferior and 2 cm medial to the femoral pulse, which is at the mid-inguinal point.
- You will feel a lump in the groin; describe as you would any lump (*see* Chapter 5, Lumps and bumps).
- A saphena varix will be smooth with a palpable thrill and will empty on minimal pressure and refill once you remove your fingers.

✔ **Perform the cough test**
- With the patient standing, place two fingers over the SFJ and ask the patient to cough; if you feel a thrill, then this suggests an incompetence of the valve.

✔ **Palpate the varicosities**
- To confirm the vascular origin of the varicosities, you can gently press on them and then release, watching them refill.
- If on doing this you elicit pain, this suggests phlebitis.
- If the veins feel hard, this may suggest thrombosis.

✔ **Palpate to check temperature**
- Gently feel with the back of your hand in the region of the varicosities; this area should normally be warm.

Special tests

These tests are used to determine the site of incompetence:

✔ **The tap test**
- Find a prominent varicosity. Place one hand over the SFJ and the other over the varicosity.
- Then tap over the SFJ; if you feel a fluid thrill transmitted to the site of the varicosity, this suggests incompetence at the SFJ.

✔ **The Trendelenburg/tourniquet test**
- This determines the level of incompetence.
- With the patient in a supine position, raise the leg to a comfortable angle for both you and the patient.

Authors' Top Tip

Do not forget to ask about hip or knee pain before you do this, as hip flexion is required to straight-leg raise!

- Hold the heel of the patient's foot with one hand (or rest it on your shoulder) and 'milk' the leg with your other hand, working proximally to drain blood from the varicosities.

- Next, apply pressure over the SFJ using a tourniquet or your fingers.
- Then ask the patient to stand and check to see if the veins refill.
  - **Veins refill immediately:** Level of incompetence is below the SFJ.
  - **Veins do not fill:** Level of incompetence is above the tourniquet, i.e. at the SFJ.
- If the initial test demonstrates incompetence below the SFJ, carry on repeating this procedure, applying the tourniquet lower and lower down the limb until you can identify the level of incompetence.
- Classically, the positions used are the mid-thigh and calf, in accordance to the lower limb venous anatomy.

✔ **Doppler probe**
- This is the most reliable of all three clinical tests for incompetence.
- Place the doppler probe over the SFJ, and with the other hand squeeze the calf, listening for the 'whoosh' sound coming from the probe.
- In a normal leg, you will only hear this noise once as the blood is forced proximally.
- In the presence of SFJ incompetence there will be a double 'whoosh'; the second is heard as the blood flows backwards through the valve when you stop squeezing the calf.
- Repeat this at the saphenopopliteal junction (SPJ).
- If provided, remember to apply ultrasound jelly to improve the acoustic window.

The Trendelenburg or the tourniquet test is essentially the same test, and indeed some examiners use the names interchangeably. The classical description of the Trendelenburg test (not to be confused with Trendelenburg's test to assess the hip abductor mechanism) involved using pressure applied by the examiner's hand rather than a tourniquet over the SFJ.

Authors' Top Tip

In actual practice we suggest you use a tourniquet rather than your hands. It is very difficult in clinical practice to apply and maintain strong enough pressure while the patient manoeuvres from the bed to stand up, let alone during finals when you will undoubtedly be very nervous; and of course you risk hurting the patient if pressing too deeply.

A tourniquet will often be provided for you, but we suggest you take your own, as in the heat of the examination you do not want to waste time working out how to lock and unlock a tourniquet that is new to you. However, in the examination you will most likely only be asked to talk about the principles of this test. In instances where the patient has valve incompetence at multiple levels, it will be difficult to interpret, and even if at the level of the SFJ the veins refill on testing, this does not necessarily mean the SFJ is competent; in fact an examiner may well ask you if you are certain it is. We suggest in this case to say that this only confirms the presence of distal incompetent perforators and that you would always confirm incompetence through the use of a hand-held doppler probe and formal venous mapping.

Authors' Top Tip

We suggest you perform the cough test after palpating for a saphena varix, as you are already ideally placed to perform this test quickly. Note that some examiners still refer to a positive cough and tap test by their eponymous names: Cruveilhier's sign and Chevrier's tap sign, respectively.

Some students may have heard of the Perthes Test, which is essentially a modification of the tourniquet test. Patients are asked to stand up and down on their tiptoes to see if their deep venous systems are non-functioning. A non-functioning deep venous system could be due to a DVT affecting vessel patency or valve incompetence. In practice, this is rarely done in undergraduate exams.

Auscultation
✔ **Auscultate over areas of multiple varicosities**
   ■ Listen for bruits, which may suggest an AvF.

Usually it is enough to simply offer to do this, as many examiners ask you to skip it.

Complete the examination
✔ **Further examination**
   ■ 'To *complete my examination, I would like to palpate for peripheral pulses and examine the abdomen, as well as perform a digital rectal examination to exclude an abdominal or pelvic mass'.*

It is important to consider secondary causes of varicose veins, particularly malignancies. Palpation of pulses is particularly important if the patient has an ulcer.

✔ **Thank the patient**
✔ **Wash your hands**
✔ **Present your findings**

Viva questions

Q1   Describe the course of the great and short saphenous vein?

(Difficult Question)

   ■ The great saphenous vein passes anterior to the medial malleolus, travels proximally in the medial aspect of the calf to the popliteal fossa and then travels along the medial aspect of the thigh to join the common femoral vein at the SFJ.
   ■ The short saphenous vein arises posterior to the lateral malleolus and ascends along the midline of the calf to join the popliteal vein in the SPJ in the popliteal fossa.

Examiner's Anecdote

'Candidates actually said the vein began at the saphenofemoral junction! I had to remind them that veins usually go towards the heart, not the other way around!'

Q2 How would you investigate this patient?
- Rule out secondary causes, e.g. abdominal/pelvic malignancies, DVT.
- Colour duplex scanning with marking of perforators.

Q3 How would you manage this patient?

(Difficult Question)

Authors' Top Tip

Remember, management involves taking a focused history to rule out secondary causes of varicose veins, a thorough clinical examination and the tailoring of investigations to your findings are needed before discussing treatment options. Always begin with these steps; however, the examiner will usually direct you to treatment options only.

Treatment can be conservative, medical or surgical.

Conservative measures include:
- Treating the underlying cause, if any, e.g. weight loss in obese patients, constipation, etc.
- Graduated compression stockings for symptomatic relief.

Surgical measures
- Injection sclerotherapy for small varicosities (e.g. sodium tetradecyl sulphate).
- Multiple stab avulsions with vein stripping and ligation of the incompetent junction (SFJ or SPJ).
- Subfascial endoscopic perforator surgery (SEPS).
- Radiofrequency or foam ablation.

Q4 What are the possible differential diagnoses?

(Difficult Question)

- Cellulitis, DVT.
- **Phlebitis:** Inflammation of superficial veins, secondary to intraluminal thrombosis; if this is migratory, it should raise suspicions about an underlying malignancy.
- Osler-Weber-Rendu syndrome (telangiectasia, recurrent epistaxis).

You will be required to know about DVT prophylaxis for surgical patients, and this may come up as part of a viva question, so be aware of the instances when prophylaxis is important. So you must say to the examiner that you will take a history to assess for the presence of risk factors such as age, OCP use, smoking, a previous history of DVT/PE and high-risk surgical procedures associated with DVT, e.g. a total knee replacement where the incidence is in excess of 50%. TED stockings and low-molecular-weight heparin are the mainstays of DVT prophylaxis.

Q5 Why is it important to check for a history of DVT in patients undergoing varicose vein surgery?

(Honours Question)

- Varicose veins may be secondary to thrombosis of the deep or superficial veins.
- If the patient's deep venous system is non-functioning, particularly after a DVT, the patient is relying on his or her superficial system for venous return.
- Varicose vein surgery will usually strip the patient's superficial veins on which they are relying.
- Such patients should therefore have doppler ultrasound scanning of their deep veins to confirm patency and check valve competence prior to surgery.
- Clinically, you could perform a Perthes test.

Q6 If the patient has an unusual rash on his or her face, what diagnosis would you consider?

(Honours Question)

- Varicose veins associated with a port wine stain and limb hypertrophy are signs seen in the rare Klippel-Trenaunay Syndrome.

Say that you would consider this diagnosis (assuming you saw the triad of signs mentioned above), particularly if the site of the varicosities didn't follow an expected anatomical pattern.

9.3 EXAMINATION OF ULCERS

There are a number of aetiologies leading to the development of ulcers that can be determined by clinical examination: they can arise as a result of arterial disease or venous insufficiency, or as a result of peripheral neuropathy, trauma or neoplastic causes, e.g. a Marjolin's ulcer (an SCC in a long-standing, non-healing ulcer) or a systemic disease leading to pyoderma gangrenosum. The majority of ulcers that you will see in clinical practice in the United Kingdom occur secondary to venous and/or arterial disease.

In finals, you may well be presented with an ulcer and asked to determine what type it is. Usually it is either venous or arterial and in some cases neuropathic.

Authors' Top Tip

Spending a day with the vascular wound care nurse would be an invaluable experience.

It will be obvious to an examiner when faced with a student who has no clear standardised method for the examination of ulcers. We suggest an examination framework that you should adopt when dealing with ulcers.

Clinical examination

Introduction
As for any clinical encounter (*see* Chapter 1, Principles of a clinical encounter). Specifically for this case:

It is acceptable at this point to ask the patient if the ulcer is painful, as this will help you work out the type of ulcer.

Inspection
✔ **General inspection of lower limbs**
  ■ Note any signs of chronic venous insufficiency, varicose veins, trophic changes, amputations or surgical scars.
✔ **Describe the site of the ulcer**
  ■ Look specifically in the following areas:

Table 9.1: Common sites of ulcers

Ulcer	Characteristic site
Arterial	Pressure areas, tips of toes
Venous	Gaiter area
Neuropathic	Heel, on the sole under the metatarsal heads

The gaiter area is the distal one third of the leg along the medial aspect, above the medial malleolus.

(Surgical Definition)

When looking at the toes for ulcers, be sure to look between the toes and at the heels; this involves manually separating the patient's toes, as well as lifting the foot to look on the underside. Warn the patient you will do this, as this may cause pain.

A neuropathic ulcer occurs typically on the sole, under the metatarsal heads.

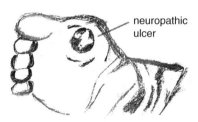

neuropathic ulcer

Figure 9.5: Neuropathic ulcer

✔ **Describe the size and shape of the ulcer**
  ■ The size of an ulcer can help differentiate the aetiology; be sure to estimate this in centimetres.
  ■ Check the shape of the ulcer to see if its margins are well defined or irregular.

Table 9.2: Size and shape of ulcers

Ulcer	Characteristic size	Characteristic shape
Arterial	Small, no larger than several centimetres	Well-defined margins with regular outline
Venous	Variable in size, but can be extremely large	Irregular outline that is variable in shape
Neuropathic	Variable, several centimetres	Regular outline

✔ **Describe the edge of the ulcer**
- Look for the following characteristic features:

Table 9.3: Ulcer edge

Ulcer	Characteristic edge
Arterial	Punched out
Venous	Sloping or flat
Neuropathic	Punched out

Other types of edges are well described in textbooks and although rare can be questioned about in a viva. For undergraduate purposes, be aware of the so-called **undermined** edge that is typical of a tuberculous ulcer; the **everted** edge seen in a malignant ulcer or the characteristic **rolled** edge in BCC. For the more ambitious student, an understanding of the pathological process that results in the different types of edge characteristics would certainly impress an examiner.

✔ **Describe the base of the ulcer**
- Estimate the depth of the ulcer; in some cases you may even see the underlying bone and tendons. If you do, say so!
- The base can demonstrate a spectrum of features, ranging from being healthy to completely avascular.
- Look for the following features and describe the base as:

Table 9.4 Ulcer base characteristics

Description	Characteristic features
Healthy	Pink granulation tissue; areas of epithelialisation
Sloughy	Offensive, exudative discharge, usually green or yellow in colour
Necrotic	Black, dead tissue
Avascular	Shiny, pale

Remember that there is a spectrum, so an ulcer may have mixed features; you can have sloughy areas with an underlying healthy granulation tissue base. This depends on the stage of healing, so we suggest you describe what you see!

Sloughy areas predispose a wound to infection, and often the wound has a discharge.

Authors' Top Tip

If you see a discharge, this should prompt you to mention to the examiner that you would take swabs for MC&S and start the patient on topical antibiotics.

An avascular floor suggests significant tissue loss and may require operative treatment with a bypass or angioplasty.

Palpation

✔ **Check if the ulcer is painful**
   ■ It is better to ask the patient this at the beginning of your examination, as you do not want to hurt the patient unduly.
   ■ No pain suggests a neuropathic ulcer, whereas a painful ulcer suggests one that is venous or arterial, although typically arterial ulcers are much more painful and require opiate analgesia.
✔ **Check the temperature of the surrounding skin**
   ■ If it is colder than the rest of the leg, consider an arterial ulcer; if it is warmer, think venous.
✔ **Check capillary refill time**
   ■ If prolonged, this suggests arterial disease and is therefore more likely to be an arterial ulcer.
✔ **Palpate the peripheral pulses (*see* Peripheral vascular examination)**
   ■ Specifically check the distal pedal pulses.

Complete the examination

✔ **Further examination**
   ■ *'To complete my examination, I would like to perform a complete peripheral vascular examination, measure the ankle brachial pressure index and complete a thorough neurological examination, looking particularly at sensation'.*
✔ **Thank the patient**
✔ **Wash your hands**
✔ **Present your findings**

The main differential for an arterial ulcer is a neuropathic ulcer. Look for other features to help distinguish between the two. Ultimately, say that you would perform a neurological examination to check sensation if you were unsure.

Table 9.5 Miscellaneous features of ulcers

Examination	Arterial	Venous	Neuropathic
Ulcer base	Necrotic, avascular, may contain slough; deep, underlying bone/tendons may be seen	Granulation tissue, sloughy	Deep, underlying bone often seen
Pain	Very painful	Painful	Painless
Temperature	Cold	Warm	Normal
Pulses	Absent	Present	Present

Viva questions

Q1   What is granulation tissue?

Granulation tissue is a heterogeneous structure that forms within the extracellular matrix at the end of the proliferative phase of wound healing. It consists of fibroblasts, macrophages and endothelial cells with a rich capillary network.

(Surgical Definition)

Q2   What is sloughy tissue?

This is moist, necrotic tissue.

(Surgical Definition)

Case 1: Venous ulcer

Instructions: Please examine the lesion on this patient's leg.

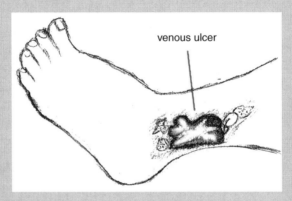

venous ulcer

Figure 9.6: Venous ulcer

Key features to look for:

Inspection

Associated paraphernalia:

- Patient may be receiving treatment for an infected ulcer, so you may see a topical antibiotic cream at the bedside.
- Also, if you see that the foot of the bed is raised, this is an important clue, as elevation is part of ulcer treatment.
- You may even see the patient's last bandage next to the bedside.

Authors' Top Tip

If you see something that may be important, it probably is! Mention it in your observation!

General inspection of the leg:
- Patient is usually an arteriopath.
- Look for signs of chronic venous insufficiency or varicose veins.

'On general inspection, the lower limbs are oedematous, with loss of hair, areas of haemo-siderin deposition and lipodermatosclerosis'.

- **Site:** found in the so-called 'gaiter area'.
- **Size/shape:** Variable in size, but can have extremely large, irregular margins.
- **Edge:** Sloping.
- **Base:** Shallow and sloughy with underlying pink granulation tissue.

Palpation
- **Temperature:** The skin surrounding the ulcer is warmer than the rest of the leg.
- Usually painless.

Completion
- Offer to examine for varicose veins as an associated feature.
- Offer ABPI; remember, an index >0.8 is a prerequisite to compression bandaging.

'I would also like to check the patient's ABPI to ensure the index is greater than 0.8, as the patient is likely to require four-layer compression bandaging as part of his treatment'.

Viva questions

Q1 What is compression bandaging?
- This is part of the treatment for venous ulcers, and most ulcers heal within a year with this treatment.

(Average Response)

- Evidence-based medicine proves that compression bandaging works, so it should be offered to all patients with an ABPI >0.8.
- An ABPI of >0.8 is important, as you want to ensure that there is no arterial component before treatment begins. Compression bandaging could compromise arterial flow to the limb.

(Good Response)

- The principle behind compression bandaging is the four-layer bandaging technique. The four layers comprise a non-adherent dressing over the actual ulcer, followed by a crepe bandage, a blue lien bandage and finally an adhesive bandage.

(Honours Response)

Examiner's Anecdote

'Candidates who actually knew there were four layers and knew what they were clearly spent time with the vascular wound care nurse and scored highly in the examination'.

Q2   **What should you consider if the ulcer fails to heal?**

(Difficult Question)

- *'The great majority of ulcers heal by 12 weeks, and most heal by a year. So if an ulcer fails to heal, I would need to consider the possibility of malignant transformation of a longstanding ulcer and arrange for a biopsy to exclude a Marjolin's ulcer'.*

Remember, as with all chronic conditions, if you are asked about management you should reply by saying you would manage the patient in a MDT management approach, with input from the wound care nurse, occupational therapists, district nurse care, etc. This demonstrates your awareness of the complexities of managing a vascular patient and gives the examiner the impression you have spent a great deal of time with actual patients in the wards.

When asked for specific treatment options, try to classify your answer into conservative and surgical measures. Under conservative measures, mention that the patient should be advised to rest and keep the limb elevated to reduce venous hypertension. Once ulcers are healed, patients should be advised to wear graduated elastic compression stockings. Although an understanding of detailed surgical treatment is not required at undergraduate level, be aware that a skin graft may be used with excision of the underlying dead skin.

Case 2: Arterial ulcer

Instructions: Please examine the lesion on this patient's foot:

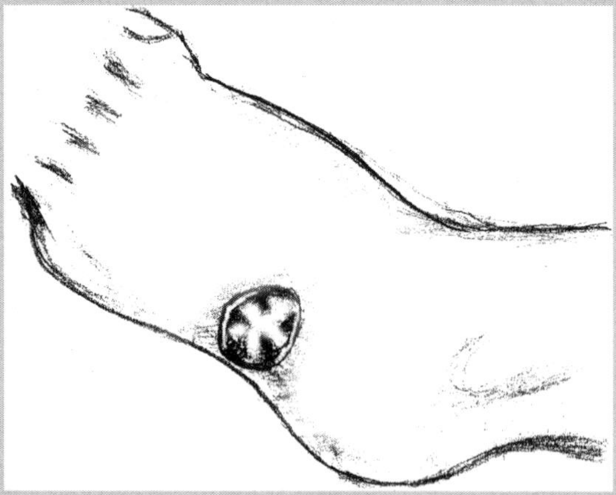

Figure 9.7: Arterial ulcer

Key features to look for:

Inspection

Associated paraphernalia:

- Patient may be on a prostaglandin infusion.

General inspection of the leg:

- Patient is usually an arteriopath.
- If the patient has an amputation of the opposite limb, then mention it.

Examiner's Anecdote

'I couldn't believe no one mentioned the patient had a below-knee amputation on the opposite leg!'

- **Site:** Usually the lesion is on the pressure areas of the feet, around the toes (especially the tips).
- **Size/shape:** Well-defined regular margin; size is variable but certainly no more than several centimetres and not as large as a venous ulcer.
- **Edge:** Characteristically punched out.
- **Base:** Absence of granulation tissue due to poor blood supply; may be necrotic or avascular; can be very deep, and in some patients you can even see tendons and bone.

'The ulcer appears deep, and I can see the underlying bone'.

Palpation

- The surrounding skin is cold and has a greyish-blue discolouration.
- There is a painful ulcer (pain may be masked by a peripheral neuropathy in diabetics).
- Peripheral pulses are absent or very difficult to feel – if you can't feel them, offer to use a doppler probe to find the most distal pulse. You are listening for the loss of the normal triphasic waveform, as seen in arteriopaths.

Completion

Treatment questions are similar to those for peripheral vascular disease (*see* Peripheral vascular examination). Pay close attention to pain relief, as arterial ulcers can be very painful. As with all questions related to pain relief, always follow the WHO analgesic ladder. The use of vasodilators such as prostaglandins or surgical techniques such as lumbar sympathectomy are beyond the scope of this book but could be a viva topic to discuss for the more ambitious student.

CHAPTER 10

Orthopaedics

Orthopaedics can bring up mixed feelings in candidates. Often this is due to a lack of time spent in an orthopaedics attachment. Some medical schools do not incorporate orthopaedics into their clinical placements, which often leads to a hit-and-miss situation. Even if you have completed a rotation in orthopaedics, we suggest as before that you set up a tutorial group with an orthopaedic registrar at the teaching hospital where you are placed. Many of the cases that will come up in finals can be seen in abundance on orthopaedics wards, and most definitely in the clinic setting.

Many patients have pain in some form or other, so always remember to be gentle and empathic with patients. Always ask before you move any joint and inform patients of what you are doing, particularly during the Special Test manoeuvres. For example, not asking about hip pain when examining a patient's knee would not sit well with the examiner or the patient, as not only does it demonstrate your lack of knowledge of referred pain, but if the patient subsequently yelped in pain, you may be penalised. Consequently, when completing any orthopaedic examination, always offer to examine the joint above and below the examination site.

Authors' Top Tip

As many of the manoeuvres in orthopaedic examinations can be daunting to a patient, ensure you give clear and simple instructions, politely demonstrating any complex manoeuvres you wish the patient to perform.

Orthopaedic examinations often follow the well-known *Look, Feel and Move* model. While this is an important structural format, it is a simplification. In addition to this, an orthopaedic examination typically involves special joint specific tests, as well as neurological and often vascular examinations of the limb involved. Most joints are also X-rayed, and this is often an important consideration when examining a patient. Therefore, do not forget to ask to look at the X-rays if appropriate.

We advocate the use of *Look, Feel and Move **plus** the 'special tests', a neurovascular examination and an X-ray* whenever you are structuring an orthopaedic examination, especially during finals.

As you will quickly come to appreciate, there is a large emphasis on observation, and we recommend if you see something you think may be an important clue, then say so. The examiners will not know you saw the wheelchair or Ilizarov frame at the bedside unless you say you saw it! Likewise, if you are examining the hip and see something else you feel may be relevant, such as a midline knee scar, then mention it!

10.1   GAIT

Gait is one of those fabled things people talk about, so we know it exists – but we never quite get to see it, especially in clinical examinations! Most candidates mention it in passing when they complete their examination. So clearly everyone knows it is important, but rarely do candidates actually examine for it. Do not be surprised if you finish early and mention you would like to examine gait that the examiner actually asks you to do so. Anything is fair game in finals.

We suggest you examine gait first, before you examine the hips or knees. This is because we believe it forms an integral part of a complete orthopaedic lower-limb examination, and by examining it first you are less likely to forget to mention it in the stress of the examination. Secondly, it falls under the *Look* or *Inspection* part of your examination, so logically should come first, and it conveniently flows onto performing a Trendelenburg Test in the hip station. Finally, an orthopaedic surgeon will be far more interested in you as a candidate after having spent an entire day watching candidates examine in exactly the same fashion; this gives you the opportunity to score brownie points.

Examiner's Anecdote

'If a student knew the different stages of gait, I would be impressed!'

Gait is actually very easy to examine, and can be very revealing. There are numerous types of pathological gait, most of which will be seen in the neurology station in medical finals; however, we will discuss the common ones you will see in surgical finals.

Authors' Top Tip

The only reason not to examine gait in a clinical setting is if you suspect a fracture, where mobilising the patient could be detrimental. As fractures are unlikely to feature in finals for obvious reasons, you won't have to worry about this.

Detailed physiology of human gait is unlikely to be a huge feature of the examination, and so only a limited understanding of the normal gait cycle will be discussed.

Remember, this is an important (albeit small) part of your lower-limb examination, so in the actual examination do not forget to introduce yourself, gain consent and perform a general inspection of the limbs before you proceed. Also, as with any musculoskeletal examination, always ask the patient if he or she has pain in the muscles, joints or back **before** performing the examination.

Clinical examination

Introduction
As for any clinical encounter (*see* Chapter 1, Principles of a clinical encounter).

Look
✔ **Check around the room for any walking aids or appliances**
  ▪ Ask if the patient can walk unaided. If he has an aid, allow him to use it. This is an important finding, particularly when presenting your examination.

e.g. *'The patient is walking unaided'* or *'The patient walks aided by a Zimmer frame'*

- Appliances could include shoe raises, orthotics or callipers. This also gives you the opportunity to score extra points by discussing walking aids early in the examination.

✔ **Ask the patient to walk**

- It is important to watch the patient walk away, turn and walk back towards you. Check for symmetry of arm swing, presence of pelvic tilt and stride length.

  e.g. *'Can you please walk several paces towards the wall, and then turn around and walk back to me?'*

✔ **Carefully observe the gait: You are looking for:**

- Presence of a limp – is the gait smooth or halted? A halted gait may be due to abductor weakness as seen in the Trendelenburg lurch, to leg shortening or to pain (antalgic gait).
- Distinctive pattern of the gait.
- The arm swing.
- How the patient turns around – can he or she turn quickly and without difficulty?

Four phases make up the gait cycle:

- Heel strike.
- Stance phase, i.e. the entire period the foot is on the ground.
- Toe off.
- Swing phase, i.e. the the foot is in the air for limb advancement.

You are unlikely to be required to know the sub-phases of the stance and swing phase. The distinctive gait pattern can help work out the cause of the patient's symptoms:

A limited or absent arm swing with the so-called shuffling gait is seen in Parkinson's disease. The patient will also find it difficult to turn around quickly and is often unstable.

Special tests: neurological pathology

✔ **Heel-to-shin test**

  e.g. *'Imagine you are on a tightrope, and walk like this…'*

✔ **Romberg's test**

  e.g. *'Please stand with your feet together like this…'* (Show the patient.) *'…and put your hands out like this'.* (Again, show the patient.)

- Explain what you plan to do, as the patient may be apprehensive that he or she may fall, which particularly in medical finals is often the case!

  e.g. *'In a minute, I'm going to ask you to close your eyes. Don't worry, I'll be standing right here to make sure you're alright. Now close your eyes for 5 to 10 seconds'.*

- **Positive test:** Patient becomes unsteady on closing the eyes; this indicates a vestibular or proprioceptive problem.

Table 10.1: Patterns of gait

Gait	Features	Pathology
Antalgic	Patient may limp and/or grimace when walking. Typically, there is a decreased stance phase and an increased swing phase.	Pain.
Trendelenburg lurch	Patient's shoulders and trunk lurch sideways in order to bring the body weight over the affected limb. Trendelenburg's test can also demonstrate this.	Weak abductors.
Drop foot	The foot 'drops' into equinus during the swing phase, and the foot is then lifted higher than normal so that the toes don't drag along the ground. The foot may slap the ground prematurely as seen in weak ankle dorsiflexors.	Peripheral neuropathy or injury to the nerves (L5) supplying the ankle dorsiflexors (common peroneal or sciatic nerve palsy).
High stepping	As above, the patient lifts the foot higher than usual, but this time, both feet are raised.	Bilateral foot drop, proprioception or cerebellar disease.
Short leg	The ipsilateral hip falls when the patient's weight bears on the short leg.	Congenital shortening, previous fracture.
Waddling	The patient's trunk moves from side to side with each step he or she takes.	Dislocation of hips, weakness of abductor muscles.

Complete the examination

Usually at this point, you would continue onto examining the lower limb, as you were originally requested.

However, if you are asked to solely examine gait, you can complete your examination by thanking the patient and asking the patient to redress. Then face the examiner and say:

✔ **Further examination**

- *'To complete my examination, I would like to perform Trendelenburg's test to check for weak hip abductors. I will measure true and apparent leg length in case the patient has a short leg gait. And I will finish by performing a complete neurological examination, looking specifically for a foot drop'.*

✔ **Thank the patient**

✔ **Wash your hands**

✔ **Present your findings, e.g.:**

'The patient appears to be comfortable and was walking unaided. She had a normal stride length, with good arm swing and was able to turn comfortably. There were no gait pattern abnormalities, and in particular there was no evidence of an antalgic or Trendelenburg's gait. In summary, these findings are consistent with a normal gait pattern'.

Viva questions

Q1 What are the different phases of gait?

(Honours Question)

- **Heel strike:** The point in the stance phase when the heel touches the ground.
- **Stance phase:** The entire period the foot is on the ground where the centre of mass acts through.
- **Toe off:** When the foot leaves the ground and the toe has terminal contact with the ground.
- **Swing phase:** The foot is in the air for limb advancement.
- Stance phase represents 60% of the gait cycle, whereas swing phase represents 40%.

Q2 What is an antalgic gait?

An antalgic gait is a gait with a decreased stance phase and increased swing phase, usually due to pain.

(Surgical Definition)

Q3 What types of walking aids are there?

(Difficult Question)

- Walking aids can be broadly classified into sticks, crutches and frames.
- There are various subtypes in each group, e.g. the Zimmer frame, elbow crutches or a wooden stick with crook handles.

Q4 Can you tell which side has the pathology from the position of the stick?

(Difficult Question)

- When using one stick, the stick should be held in the opposite hand to the side of the pathology.

Remember, you can make an intelligent guess as to which limb has the pathology by observing in which hand the patient holds the walking stick. In hip pathology, the stick is held in the opposite hand in order to reduce the weight-bearing load through the affected hip. In knee pathology, it is usually held in the ipsilateral hand (*see* Knee).

10.2 HIP

The hip is perhaps the most common case to be seen in an orthopaedic bay in finals. It would be foolish not to have a thorough understanding of its clinical examination. Candidates are often very good at examining the hip, and as such the better candidates will need to demonstrate an edge when confronted with this case.

Clinical examination

Introduction

As for any clinical encounter (*see* Chapter 1, Principles of a clinical encounter).

Look

✔ **Check around the room for any walking aids or appliances**
✔ **Observe the patient from the front**
- Check the level of the hips and knees; are they symmetrical?

- Look for any obvious valgus/varus deformity of knees.
- Look for any surgical scars. (If the patient has a vertical knee scar, then mention it; he or she may have OA in the hips and knees!).
- Is there an obvious leg length discrepancy?

✔ **Observe the patient from the back**
  - Look for any surgical scars (checking the posterior approach to the hip).
  - Is there gluteal muscle wasting?
  - Is there a scoliosis (*see* Back)?

A compensatory scoliosis can be seen in true shortening. Patients may even have a shoe raise, hence the importance of checking for any walking aids early in the examination!

✔ **Examine the gait (*see* Gait)**
✔ **Perform Trendelenburg's test**

There are many variations in performing this test. Some candidates like to sit on a chair or kneel on the ground with their hands placed on the patient's hips and the patient's arms on the candidate's shoulders for support. Some like to stand and hold the patient's arms and simply observe the patient's hips. We suggest you do what you are most familiar and comfortable with in the examination.

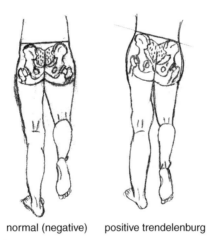

normal (negative)   positive trendelenburg

Figure 10.1: Trendelenburg's test

- Offer the patient support, as patients are often afraid they may fall.
- Ask the patient to raise one leg and hold it for some time; watch what happens to the hips.

Authors' Top Tip

It often helps to demonstrate this to the patient, as some patients may straight-leg raise instead of flexing the hip and knee joint.

- **Positive test:** The ipsilateral hip falls.
- Repeat with the opposite leg.

Closer inspection:

✔ Measure leg length

This clearly means you should bring a measuring tape with you to the examination. We suggest the automatic roll-up type, as you don't want to have to unknot a tape in the examination. In most cases, however, the examiner will tell you to skip this and carry on.

- Do a quick screen by looking to see if the levels of the hips, knees and ankles are symmetrical. Often, looking at the ankles offers the best clue for any leg length discrepancy.
- **First measure apparent leg length:** This means measuring from any fixed anatomical point (classically the xiphisternum) to the medial malleolus. (We suggest using the umbilicus as the anatomical point of reference.)
- **Then measure true leg length:** This means measuring from the anterior superior iliac spine (ASIS) to the medial malleolus.
  - If there is shortening on either side, you need to decide if it's at the level of the knees or above (the Galeazzi test).
  - Compare the level of the knees to see if the shortening is femoral or tibial in origin.
  - Flex both knees to 90°. Look horizontally to see if one knee is shorter.
  - If the shortening is above the knee, consider femoral shortening; below is tibial.
  - If the shortening is above the knee, then approximate the distance between the ASIS and the greater trochanter. Is there a difference on either side? If there is, this suggests that the shortening is within the hip joint itself.

Feel

✔ **Palpate over bony landmarks for tenderness**
- Palpate over the ASIS, PSIS and the greater trochanter for tenderness.
- Pain over the greater trochanter may indicate trochanteric bursitis.

Move

Always check active movements before passive, estimate range of movement, and compare both sides.

✔ **Check hip flexion (130°)**

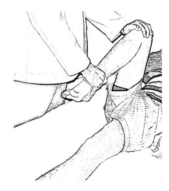

Figure 10.2: Hip flexion

- Flex the knee and hold it, then flex the hip and move the knee right up to the patient's chest.
- Remember to watch the pelvis, focusing on the ASIS. As soon as the pelvis begins to move, the hip is no longer flexing, and the pelvis is moving, i.e. the range of true hip flexion has been reached.

✔ **Check abduction (45°) and adduction (30°)**

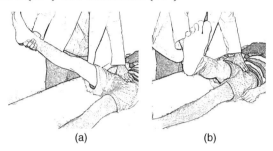

(a)   (b)

Figure 10.3: (a) Hip abduction; (b) Hip adduction

- Stabilise the pelvis by placing one arm across the ASIS.

Authors' Top Tip

Most textbooks say to use your left hand to stabilise the pelvis; frankly, we have never seen a hand big enough to reach across both anterior superior iliac spines!

- With the free hand, hold the patient's ankle, then abduct and adduct the leg over the other leg until you feel the pelvis starting to move.

✔ **Check rotation (internal 35° and external 45°)**

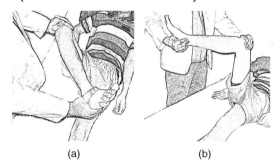

(a)   (b)

Figure 10.4: (a) Hip internal rotation; (b) Hip external rotation

- Move to the end of the bed, and gently cradle both ankles in either hand internally, then externally rotate both legs.
- You are looking to see the range of movement of the patella (as a reference point).
- An alternative method involves flexing both the hip and knees to 90° then internally and externally rotating the hip joint; then repeating with the opposite leg.

✔ **Check hip extension (10°)**

- This is easiest done if the patient is asked to lie in the lateral position.
- If the patient is in the left lateral position, extend the right hip outwards, and vice versa.

Special tests

✔ **Perform Thomas' test**

A fixed flexion deformity can be masked by a lumbar lordosis; Thomas' test checks for a fixed flexion deformity.

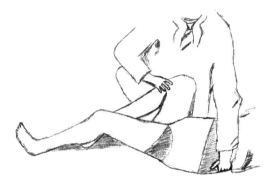

Figure 10.5: Fixed flexion deformity of the left knee

- Place your left hand in the left hollow of the patient's lumbar spine (the patient's knees will be in a neutral position at 90°).
- With your other hand, flex the hip and knee of the **opposite** leg until the lumbar spine straightens against your hand (the range of flexion of the opposite hip is normally 130°).
- Then extend the ipsilateral leg until straight; in normal patients, it should straighten completely, if the patient has a fixed flexion deformity, you will see flexion of the fixed knee.

Complete the examination

✔ **Further examination**

- *'To complete my examination, I would like to assess the **neurovascular status** of the lower limbs and examine the knees and back'.*
- If you felt there was pathology, you can ask to see the X-rays at this point; if not, then offer to look at the X-rays when presenting your findings.

Always examine the neurology, the vascular supply as well as the joint above and below, as pain can be referred.

✔ **Thank the patient**

✔ **Wash your hands**

✔ **Present your findings:** Turn to the examiner and maintain eye contact; some candidates start fidgeting with their hands–if it helps, fold your hands behind your back.

Examiner's Anecdote

'It is annoying when candidates constantly look back at the patient, as if the patient will reveal some new information! The candidate is presenting to me, so I expect the candidate to be looking at me!'

Case 1: Osteoarthritis of the hips

Instructions: Please examine this patient's hip.

Key features to look for:

Look

- Patient is usually >50 years old.
- **Functional aids:** Walking aids, especially a walking stick (with the stick held in the hand opposite to the affected hip; this is to reduce impact load in the affected hip).
- **Gait:** An obvious limp, an antalgic gait or a Trendelenburg's gait.
- **Trendelenburg's test:** Positive.
- **From the front:** A hip scar is often seen in the opposite hip (patients are usually awaiting an arthroplasty for the other hip), muscle wasting, leg length discrepancy.
- **From the back:** Lumbar lordosis may be increased in those with a fixed flexion deformity, scoliosis, scars from a posterior approach.

Closer inspection

- Affected leg will appear short (as hip is adducted with the leg in external rotation).
- Fixed flexion deformity (this may only be seen with Thomas' test).

Feel: Tenderness.

Move: Movements are generally restricted.

Special tests: Thomas' test demonstrates a fixed flexion deformity.

Viva questions

Q1 What does a positive Trendelenburg test indicate?
- Weakness of the hip abductors.

(Average Response)

- There are many causes of a positive Trendelenburg test:
  - This could be a false positive, usually due to pain or poor balance on the patient's part as a result of generalised weakness.
  - Gluteal muscle inhibition due to pain from the hip joint.
  - Gluteal muscle inefficiency due to a congenital hip dislocation or coxa vara.
  - Gluteal muscle paralysis from polio.

(Good Response)

Q2 How would you investigate this patient?
- *'I would like to perform* **simple blood tests** *such as renal function tests, as the patient is likely to be on long-term NSAIDs, which may lead to interstitial nephritis.*
- *I would also like to request* **specialist blood tests,** *particularly Rheumatoid factor and ANA, to exclude a systemic cause.*

- *I would also request **imaging,** which would include plain-film radiographs of the affected hip with two views, AP and lateral, and views of the joint above and below'.*

(Good Response)

Q3 What radiological features you would expect to find in an osteoarthritic hip?
- Loss of joint space.
- Osteophytes.
- Sclerosis.
- Subchondral cysts.

Loss of articular cartilage is an early sign, with osteophytes at joint edges seen later in the disease process.

Q4 What radiological features would you expect to find in rheumatoid arthritis?

(Difficult Question)

- Periarticular osteoporosis.
- Loss of joint space.
- Marginal erosions.
- Absence of osteophytes.

Q5 How would you treat OA?
- *'The management of OA involves a **multidisciplinary team management** approach with input from orthopaedic surgeons and the GP, physiotherapist and occupational therapist.*
- *But in general it can be divided into conservative, medical and surgical measures'.*

Conservative measures involve:
- Lifestyle changes, particularly functional aids to help with daily living activities, such as dressing.
- A walking stick held in the opposite hand to aid mobility.
- Avoiding activities that would increase impact loading in the affected hip, such as walking uphill.
- Weight loss and regular physiotherapy.

Medical treatments involve:
- Pain relief via adoption of the WHO analgesic ladder.
- Particularly the use of paracetamol as first line, with anti-inflammatories targeting COX-1 and 2 receptors (rofecoxib) and prophylactic peptic ulcer medication.

Surgical interventions:
- These vary according to the age of the patient, but in general if the patient is >50 years old, a total joint replacement is the procedure of choice.
- As younger patients have at least one revision in their lifetime, they benefit from other procedures such as a repositioning osteotomy until an arthroplasty becomes a viable option.

(Honours Response)

Q6   What features would suggest that a total joint replacement be suitable?

(Difficult Question)

- Intractable pain (with failure of conservative and medical measures).
- Rest pain, instability or loss of mobility.

Q7   What would you expect to find in a hip affected by rheumatoid arthritis?

(Difficult Question)

- The patient usually has an established pattern of multiple joint involvement that is typically symmetrical.
- There is marked gluteal muscle and calf wasting.
- The affected limb is held in fixed flexion in external rotation.
- All movements are generally restricted and painful. whereas in OA the movements may be restricted but are often painless within a limited range.

10.3   KNEE

The knee is the largest joint and supports the entire weight of the human body, making it vulnerable to both acute injury and osteoarthritis. It is also the second-most common case to come up in an orthopaedics bay in finals. Acute injuries are unlikely to be present in finals but can form a basis for discussion in the viva. Common conditions to affect the knee that you must read about prior to the examination include RA, OA and soft tissue injuries.

Clinical examination

Introduction
As for any clinical encounter (*see* Chapter 1, Principles of a clinical encounter).

Look
✔ **Check around the room for any walking aids or appliances**
✔ **Observe the knee**

Be sure to observe the knee from the front and the back for:
- **Symmetry:** Comment on symmetry of the patella, equal shape and height or the presence of lumpy knees (osteophytes).
- **Deformities:** Assess knee alignment for:
  - 'Bow legs' (genu varum), most commonly seen in OA and Paget's disease.
  - 'Knock knees' (genu valgum), seen in adults suffering from RA.
  - Deformities of the foot that can contribute to knee pathology, such as high-arched feet (pes cavus) or flat feet (pes planus).
- **Swellings:**
  - Swelling could be a localised effusion that may be reactive or secondary to OA; haemarthrosis (commonly associated with tibial plateau fractures, which are difficult to see on X-ray); or septic arthritis, which is diagnosed with aspiration of the fluid and tested for MC&S and Gram stain.
  - Prepatellar bursitis (housemaid's knee); infrapatellar bursitis (clergyman's knee).

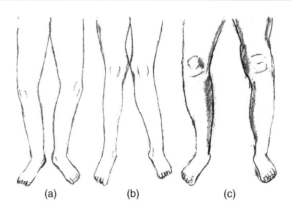

(a)   (b)   (c)

Figure 10.6: (a) Genu varum; (b) Valgus; (c) right Paget's knee

    – Extending beyond the synovial cavity (as a result of injury, long bone infection, tumour).
    – Popliteal fossa swellings (e.g. Baker's cyst).
- **Scars:** Anterior midline (used commonly in TKR), posterior midline (access to the popliteal fossa) or small, barely visible scars from arthroscopic access points.
- **Skin appearance:** Erythematous, suggesting localised infection; bruising as a result of trauma.
- **Quadriceps muscle wasting:** Wasting or loss of bulk is related to the muscle not being used, which may occur as a result of a painful knee (related to trauma or infection, OA, RA, etc). Officially this is tested by measuring the circumference and comparing it with that of the other leg. Offer to measure at this point in the examination. Measure thigh circumference 10 cm proximal to the upper pole of the patella, which corresponds to the position of the vastus medialis muscle.

✔ Examine gait (*see* Section 10.1)

Feel

✔ **Temperature**
- Is the knee warm to the touch? This could be a sign of infection or part of an inflammatory response, as seen in RA, tumours and trauma to the knee.

✔ **Tenderness**
- **Palpate the joint line:** Begin by flexing the knee joint and palpating along the joint line, identifying the borders of the femur and tibia, then palpate around the entire joint line, identifying areas of localised tenderness.
- <u>Look for:</u> Tenderness over the medial end of the tibial tubercle, which suggests medial meniscal damage, or in the adolescent patient, evidence of Osgood-Schlatter's disease. You would expect widespread tenderness in septic arthritis.

Authors' Top Tip

Candidates may have heard of the Apley's grind test and Clark's test. We recommend you do not attempt these, as positive results are indicated by pain. A patient in pain will certainly make you lose valuable points.

✔ **Effusion**

This occurs most commonly as a result of trauma or infection irritating the lining of the knee joint. The presence of an effusion can be assessed with the following tests:

- **Patella tap test:** To perform, you will need to use both hands. Place the fingertips of the first hand on the patella, and with the thumb and index finger of the second hand, milk any fluid present in the suprapatellar pouch down to the superior tip of the patella, starting at approximately 15 cm superiorly.
  - If positive, the patella will move up and down on the fluid.
  - If there is only a small effusion, the patellar tap test will be negative, in which case employ the Stroke test.
- **Stroke test:** This is explained most easily in three steps:
  - Empty the suprapatellar pouch using the thumb and index finger of one hand, as described above in the patellar tap test.
  - Massage from the medial side of the knee joint, forcing the fluid laterally.
  - Now, watch the medial side whilst you gently massage from the lateral surface of the joint, as this will bulge in the presence of an effusion.
- Both of these tests will be negative in the presence of a tense effusion.

In actual fact, there are a range of clinical tests that can be used to detect the presence of fluid. The amount of fluid in the knee will determine which test is best suited. However, it is sufficient to know the above two tests for undergraduate level. Be aware that the stroke test is also known as the 'bulge' or 'fluid displacement' test.

Move

Always check active movements before passive, and estimate the range of movement in degrees, comparing both sides.

✔ **Assess extensor apparatus**
- Assess the integrity of the Quadriceps muscle.
- Ask the patient to straight-leg raise; if you notice the knee bending as the leg is raised, this suggests either a fixed flexion deformity or weakness of the quadriceps group of muscles.
- In order to differentiate between the two causes:
  - Take the weight of the leg in your examining hand and passively straight-leg raise.
  - If the knee joint remains flexed as you straight-leg raise, this suggests a fixed flexion deformity (and is usually due to arthritic changes).
  - If the knee joint straightens, then the initial knee flexion that was seen on active straight-leg raise is a result of quadriceps muscle weakness.

✔ **Assess knee flexion**
- Passively flex the knee joint, placing one of your hands on the patellar surface to feel for crepitus (this has a crunchy feel) with movement, indicating changes at the articular surface.
- Measure the degree of flexion at the joint (normally >135°); a reduction in flexion may be secondary to OA changes or the presence of an effusion at the joint.

✔ **Assess knee extension**

- Passively extend the knee, feeling for crepitus and checking for the presence of hyperextension (*genu recurvatum*).
- The range of movement should normally be 0°. Hyperextension may signify instability of the joint.

Special tests

There are several tests that assess the integrity of the ligaments and check for meniscal tears.

Authors' Top Tip
Mention to the examiner that if this is very painful for the patient, EUA should be considered.

✔ **Assess the collateral ligaments**

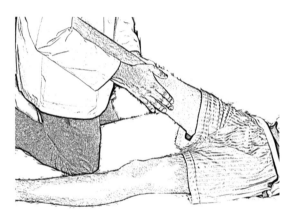

Figure 10.7: Collateral ligament stress test

- Test by flexing the knee to 20° (this is very important, as it prevents the knee locking in extension).
- **Medial collateral:** Place your right hand on the lateral surface of the knee (this will provide stability), and using your free hand hold just above the medial meniscus and abduct the leg. If the leg goes into valgus, this is highly suggestive of a medial collateral rupture; if the degree of valgus is severe, then one needs to consider the possibility of a posterior cruciate rupture in addition to a rupture of the medial collateral ligament.
- **Lateral collateral:** This time, use your right hand to provide support and place it on the medial side of the knee; using the left hand placed superiorly to the lateral malleolus, adduct the leg. If the leg goes into varus, this suggests a tear of the lateral collateral ligament; if the degree of varus is severe, then there is probably a coinciding rupture of the posterior cruciate ligament.
- Don't forget to compare both sides!

✔ **Assess the cruciate ligaments**

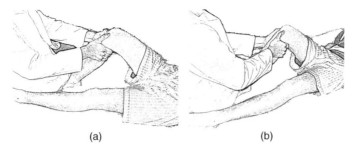

(a)   (b)

Figure 10.8: (a) Anterior drawer test; (b) Posterior drawer test

- **Anterior and posterior drawer tests:** This is done with the knee flexed to 90° and the hip at 45°.
  - First, inspect the alignment of the femur and tibia from the side; if the tibia is not aligned and is displaced inferiorly to the femur, one can assume that there is a tear of the posterior collateral.
  - Next, you must anchor the foot down; this can be done by lightly sitting on it.
  - Now grasp the lower leg at the superior end of the tibia (just below the tibial tubercle) firmly on both sides. This is best done by wrapping your fingers posteriorly around the leg with the thumbs placed on the anterior surface.
  - After ensuring the patient is relaxed, perform the **posterior drawer test** by pushing the leg away from you, thereby testing the integrity of the PCL.
  - Then perform the **anterior drawer test** by pulling the leg towards you, this time testing for the integrity of the ACL.
  - If the knee is displaced anteriorly, i.e. a positive anterior draw test – and by greater than 1.5 cm – then this most definitely suggests a rupture of the ACL (often in association with rupture of the medial collateral ligament).
  - If you noted a posterior sag initially (>1 cm), this suggests damage to the PCL; in this case, be careful, as you may get a false positive anterior draw test. This is because the perceived extra anterior movement would simply be related to reducing the initial posterior sag.
- **The Lachman test:**
  - This sensitive test also checks for ACL instability.

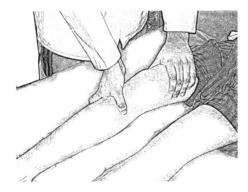

Figure 10.9: Lachman test

- – Here the leg is flexed to 30° only. One hand is placed on the femur just above the knee joint to provide stability, and the other hand is placed proximally on the tibia with the fingers wrapped posteriorly and the thumb anteriorly just above the tibial tuberosity, then pulled upwards towards you.
- – If it gives, then this is regarded as being positive for an ACL rupture.

There are other special tests that can be done to assess knee pathology, but most are too painful to be performed in a clinical examination. The Pivot shift test, which is another test used to assess the ACL, is best done under anaesthesia, as it is very painful. The patellar apprehension test is also best avoided.

To assess the menisci, it is often enough in finals to have palpated the joint line during the Feel part of your knee examination, checking for tenderness or oedema in the joint line, which would suggest meniscal damage. McMurray's test is done to help differentiate between medial and lateral meniscal tears. However, as the test adds little to the actual examination and is painful, you will not normally be required to carry this out during your examination. However, you may be asked to describe the principles of the test (*see* Viva Q1).

Complete the examination

✔ **Further examination**

- ■ *'To complete my examination, I would like to examine the hip and the ankles. I would also like to perform a complete lower limb neurovascular exam'.*
- ■ If you feel there is pathology, you can ask to see the X-rays at this point; if not, then offer to look at the X-rays when presenting your findings.

The popliteal, posterior tibial and dorsalis pedis pulses are important peripheral pulses to feel. You may note a popliteal aneurysm, which would feel pulsatile and expansile, or a popliteal cyst also known as a Baker's cyst; this is a non-tender, fluctuant lump. In the absence of peripheral pulses but in the presence of a popliteal pulse, this may suggest an occlusion.

If you wish to look at the X-rays, be sure to request weight-bearing X-rays with at least two views: AP and lateral.

✔ **Thank the patient**
✔ **Wash your hands**
✔ **Present your findings**

Viva questions

Q1   How would you perform McMurray's Test?

(Difficult Question)

- ■ The opposite leg to the one being tested should be placed in a position of abduction; the leg being tested is then flexed at the hip joint with the knee held at 90°.
- ■ Place your left hand over the kneecap and your thumb and index fingers at the inferior joint line of the knee.

- Then, with the foot held in external rotation, extend the leg with your right hand and watch the patient's face for pain; if you feel a click at the medial meniscus, this suggests a tear of the medial meniscus.
- For the lateral meniscus, repeat the above test but this time with the foot held in internal rotation; pain plus a click suggests a tear of the lateral meniscus.
- It is important to note that when performing the above manoeuvres, to be considered a true McMurray's test, the application of both a varus and valgus force is necessary; this is because the results would be otherwise adversely affected.

Q2   What provides stability to the knee joint?

(Difficult Question)

- The following ligaments, as described below:
    - The ACL and PCL (intracapsular), as the names suggest, stop the tibia moving anteriorly and posteriorly respectively in relation to the femur.
    - The medial and lateral collateral ligaments (extracapsular) provide support for the capsule of the knee.
    - The medial collateral is attached to the medial tibial condyle and protects against a valgus force.
    - The lateral collateral is attached to the head of the fibula and protects against a varus force.
- And the following muscles, as described below:
    - The quadriceps and hamstring are massive providers of stability to the knee joint.
    - It is this fact that negates the need for ACL or PCL reconstruction and is also the reason patients are sent for quadriceps and hamstring exercises alone in such cases, as these muscles can compensate for the stability required.

Q3   What is the purpose of the fibula?

(Difficult Question)

- It acts as a support for the tibia, so in lower-limb fractures if only the tibia is fractured, it can be treated in plaster alone, as it is considered to be a relatively stable injury.
- When both the tibia and fibula are fractured, then most centres treat with an intramedullary nail of the tibia, as this is classified as an unstable fracture.

Case 1: Osteoarthritis of the knee

Instructions: Please examine this patient's knee.

Key features to look for:

Look
- A walking stick.
- Varus deformity; fixed-flexion deformity.

- Opposite knee having a midline scar, indicating previous TKR.
- Quadriceps muscle wasting.
- Antalgic gait.

Feel

- There may be joint line tenderness.
- An effusion may be present.

Move

- Crepitus on movement.
- Decreased range of flexion.
- Fixed-flexion deformity of the knee may become apparent.
- Generalised tenderness on active and passive movement.

Special tests: Positive McMurray's Test.

Completion

Viva questions

Q1 What features would you look for in X-ray?
- *'This patient is likely to have OA of the knee.*
- *I would request weight-bearing X-rays of the knee, with AP and lateral views looking specifically for: Loss of joint space, Osteophytes, Sclerosis and Subchondral cysts'.*

(Good Response)

OA changes are best remembered using the infamous mnemonic 'LOSS'. You may see chondrocalcinosis on X-rays; these are soft tissue calcifications in the joint. Weight bearing is essential, as this can demonstrate varying levels of articular cartilage thinning.

Q2 How would you manage OA of the knee?
For a detailed answer (*see* Gait, Case 1: Viva Q5). OA knee is essentially managed in a similar fashion using an MDT management approach. Details specific to the knee include:

- Physiotherapy to improve quadriceps muscle strength.
- Simple analgesia in the form of paracetamol or co-codamol.
- Walking aids in the form of sticks or frames.
- Intra-articular steroid injection for temporary pain relief.
- Partial or total knee arthroplasty.

OA of the knees is the most common knee case you will see in finals. RA of the knee is less likely, but quiescent arthritis has been seen in finals before. It would be difficult to distinguish between the two at this stage in your medical careers on clinical examination alone. However, be able to compare X-ray findings in both OA and RA. The absence of osteophytes is a key distinguishing feature. For X-ray changes in RA (*see* Section 10.1, Case 1: Viva Q4).

10.4 FOOT AND ANKLE

Although uncommon in the orthopaedics section of finals, foot and ankle examinations have come up before and indeed came up in the finals of one of the authors. So be prepared for anything. When feet and ankles do appear in finals, often it's as a short case. Nonetheless, a complete examination will be described. The vast majority of candidates will not have even examined an ankle or foot prior to finals, and so by preparing you are already at an advantage. A&E Minors offers an excellent opportunity to examine ankles and feet, but more often than not these are sprains and fractures, which are unlikely to appear in finals.

Clinical examination

Introduction

As for any clinical encounter (*see* Chapter 1, Principles of a clinical encounter).

Look

✔ **Check around the room for any walking aids or appliances**
- If you see any, mention them.
- This can lead onto a discussion about walking aids (*see* Gait).

✔ **Examine the patient's shoes**

Authors' Top Tip

This may seem odd to most candidates, but you can learn a lot from the patient's shoes. In fact, the orthopaedic consultant would be impressed if you asked to look at the patient's shoes, let alone know what you are looking for!

- If the shoe is custom made or is an orthopaedic device, then mention it, e.g. '*The patient appears to have Piedro® boots'.*
- Look for any orthotic devices, e.g. drop foot splints, calipers.
- Check inside the shoes for any moulded insoles.
- Look at the soles for any abnormal wear patterns or any elevation of the soles or shoe heels.

✔ **Observe the patient while standing**
- Check the patient's posture. Is he or she slouching?
- Does the patient show any signs of pain when standing, e.g. grimacing?
- Take a gross look for any scars or swellings.
- Look with the patient's feet together, as it may be easier to spot a varus or valgus abnormality of the knees.
- Check for the **normal** varus of the heels from behind by asking the patient to stand on his or her tiptoes.

✔ **Examine the gait**
- Look for patterns, such as an antalgic gait, a foot droop or a high-stepping gait.
- Specifically you are looking for a normal heel strike, a toe-off phase and if the foot is flat during the stance phase (plantigrade).

- Other less-common features you may see include:
  - High-stepping gait due to a fixed equinis deformity.
  - Foot that is inverted and supinated during walking due to *hallux rigidus*.
  - The so-called 'peg leg' seen in talipes calcaneus.

✔ **Observe the patient while sitting**

Some candidates prefer to sit while the patient places his or her foot in the candidate's lap. Others prefer the patient to sit while manoeuvring the patient's foot as required.

- **Inspect the forefoot:** Look at the longitudinal arch for flattening (*pes planus*) or if the arch is high (*pes cavus*).
- **Inspect the toes:** Look specifically at the big toe for *hallux valgus* or *rigidus*. Examine the lesser toes for hammer, claw or mallet deformities.
  e.g. *'There is a significant hallux valgus deformity of the left great toe, with overriding of the second toe and an associated bunion'.*
- **Inspect the nails** for changes, e.g. psoriasis or onychogryphosis.
- **Inspect the sole** for callosities or bunions.
- **Inspect the hindfoot:** Look at the heel for any hindfoot deformities, e.g. valgus or varus.

Feel

✔ **Check temperature**
- Is there any temperature difference, e.g. a warm foot, as in septic arthritis?

✔ **Palpate for tenderness**
- Palpate the hindfoot, midfoot, forefoot and around the joint line from medial to lateral malleolus.
- **Specific sites for palpation:** Base of the fifth metatarsal (MT), the first MTPJ, the base of the first tarsometatarsal joint, and the navicular tubercle.
- Feel for joint crepitations.

✔ **Palpate the Achilles tendon**
- First, feel for any obvious defects.
- Ask the patient to stand on tiptoes and palpate again, feeling for a palpable gap.
- You can perform Simmonds' test if appropriate (*see* Special tests).

Move

✔ **Check ankle joint movements**
- Isolate the joint first, e.g. if examining the right ankle, cup the distal tibia (shin) with your left hand; with your right hand, grip the heel (the patient's soles should rest against your forearm).
- Using your right hand and right forearm, dorsi and plantarflex the ankle.
- Dorsiflexion (20°) and plantarflexion (40°).

✔ **Check subtalar joint movements**
- Isolate by holding the heel in your left hand and gripping the talus in the right hand.
- With your right hand, **evert** (20°) and **invert** (10°) the foot.

✔ **Check midtarsal joint (forefoot) movements**
- Isolate by holding the ankle still, with the left hand gripping the heel.

- With your right hand, hold the forefoot.
- Moving the tarsus, first abduct and adduct the forefoot, then plantar and dorsiflex.

✔ **Check MTPJ movements**
  - Isolate by holding the forefoot with the left hand just proximal to the MTPJ.
  - With the right hand, dorsi and plantarflex the MTPJ of the big toe and the subsequent lesser toes.
  - Check for extension of all toes simultaneously by moving all toes in one movement: *'Can you please curl your toes for me?'*

Special tests

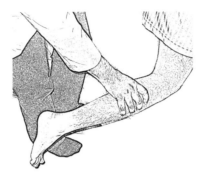

Figure 10.10: Simmonds' test

✔ **Calf squeeze test (Simmonds' test)**
  - Palpate the Achilles tendon up to the gastrocnemius. Feel for any defects in the tendon or swelling or tenderness along this path.
  - With the patient lying prone or kneeling on the couch, squeeze the calf distal to its largest diameter.
  - If it is normal, you should see plantarflexion of the foot. If this is absent, it suggests tendon rupture.

Authors' Top Tip

Before squeezing the calf, some candidates prefer to position the patient kneeling on a chair or the examining couch with the patient's foot hanging over the bed. This is an acceptable alternative.

Complete the examination

✔ **Further examination**
  - *'To complete my examination I would like to perform a complete neurological and vascular examination of the lower limbs, as well as examine the joint above and below'.*
✔ **Thank the patient**
✔ **Wash your hands**
✔ **Present your findings**

Note that there are several tests to check ankle joint stability and/or ligamentous injuries. This is not required for undergraduate examinations. These injuries are usually associated with fractures and can cause considerable pain, thus examination is reserved only for clinical need and performed under anaesthesia. You are likely to see such patients in A&E Minors; they will usually be inhaling nitrous oxide from a tank of Entonox, with impressive bruising over the ankle joint.

Viva questions

Q1   What are hammer toes, mallet toes and claw toes?

(Difficult Question)

- These are common deformities of the lesser toes.
- **Hammer toes:** This is a flexion deformity of the proximal interphalangeal joint (PIPJ) with the distal interphalangeal joint (DIPJ) commonly in extension.
- **Mallet toes:** This is a flexion deformity of the DIPJ.
- **Claw toes:** This is a flexion deformity of the PIPJ and the DIPJ.

Management in general involves the use of appropriate footwear (except in mallet toes) and operative measures. In all cases, the deformity can be fixed or mobile. This is an important consideration, as this determines the surgical options available. All these conditions are more commonly found in women, those with RA and the elderly. They are caused by an imbalance between the extrinsic and intrinsic muscles of the lesser toes.

Q2   What are the causes of pain in the forefoot?

(Honours Question)

Forefoot pain is known as metatarsalgia. In theory, any foot abnormality can cause metatarsalgia due to uneven weight distributions, so it can be seen in *hallux valgus*, flat foot, etc. There are specific conditions to the forefoot that are worth knowing about, albeit briefly, for finals.

- **Stress fracture:** Also known as a march fracture of the second and third metatarsal bones after unaccustomed exercise, as seen in e.g. marathon runners or new army recruits. Initial X-rays are normal, therefore patients should be X-rayed again 2 weeks later. Treatment is rest.
- **Morton's neuroma:** Localised tenderness in the third intermetatarsal space. Patients typically complain of forefoot pain radiating to the toes. The condition leads to the impression of digital nerve entrapment, secondary to nerve thickening. It usually responds to a change to appropriate footwear, but refractory cases may need excision.
- **Frieberg's disease:** This is osteochondritis of the second metatarsal head. Treatment is with appropriate footwear and surgery.

Case 1: *Hallux valgus*

Instructions: Please examine this woman's foot.

Key features to look for:
Look
- An obvious valgus deformity of the great toe; estimate degree of valgus if possible

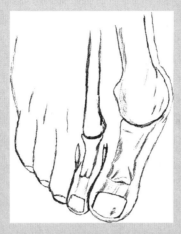

Figure 10.11: Hallux valgus

- Usually bilateral.
- There is also usually an associated bunion over the medial aspect of the first metatarsal head.
- Callosities over the soles.
- The shoes will have a normal weight-bearing wear pattern.

<u>Feel:</u> Tenderness over the first MTPJ
<u>Move:</u> Hypermobility of the first MTPJ

Completion
Request to see weight-bearing X-rays to accurately measure the degree of valgus deformity and to look for the presence of OA of the first MTPJ. Accurate calculation of the so-called intermetatarsal angle from the X-rays can help guide operative treatment with an osteotomy in the non-arthritic patient.

Viva questions

Q1 What causes *hallux valgus*?
- It is idiopathic and familial.
- The long-term use of shoes, particularly narrow, pointy shoes and high heels, can cause this.
- It can be associated with RA.

Q2 How would you treat *hallux valgus*?

(Difficult Question)

Conservative measures include:
- The use of appropriate shoes, i.e. those with wide toe boxes, protective padding and no heel.
- Physiotherapy and OT if necessary.

Surgical measures include:

- Realignment osteotomy.
- Excision arthroplasty or fusion.
- Surgical excision of the bunion.

Q3 What do you know of *hallux rigidus*?

(Honours Question)

- There is an inability to dorsiflex the first MTPJ due to pain.
- This degenerative joint disease is usually due to OA or gout.
- Clinically patients have pain in the first MTPJ and will complain of pain when walking. This will be evident on examination of the gait during the push-off phase.
- Patients can be managed conservatively with appropriate shoes, such as the 'rocker bottom' shoe to aid dorsiflexion.

10.5 SHOULDER

The shoulder is a ball-and-socket type of joint; it is the most mobile joint in the body. Its range of motion is possible due to the number of bones, joints, muscles, tendons and ligaments present. The shoulder joint consists of three bones: the humerus, the scapula and the clavicle. It is the articulations between these bones that make up the joints of the shoulder: the acromioclavicular, the sternoclavicular and the glenohumeral joints. The glenohumeral joint is most commonly known as the shoulder joint.

The muscles that contribute to the stability and movements at the shoulder joint consist of the deltoid and teres major muscles, in combination with a group of muscles known collectively as the rotator cuff muscles. All these muscles originate from the scapula and insert onto the head of the humerus. Be aware of the function of each muscle at the shoulder joint, as you may well be asked this in the viva!

Table 10.2: Shoulder muscles

Muscle	Action
Deltoid	Abduction, flexion and extension
Teres major	Medial rotation of humerus and adduction
Supraspinatus	Abduction
Infraspinatus	External rotation
Teres minor	External rotation
Subscapularis	Internal rotation

If you are asked to examine a shoulder in finals, you are likely to be dealing with: rotator cuff tendinitis, frozen shoulder, a cuff tear or a recurrent shoulder dislocation with instability. Winging of the scapula may turn up as a spot diagnosis. However, as repeated examinations can be painful, you may see a patient who has had operative treatment for his or her condition. You may therefore be quizzed on the principles behind these various conditions.

Introduction
As for any clinical encounter (*see* Chapter 1, Principles of a clinical encounter).

Look
This needs to be done anteriorly, posteriorly, laterally and superiorly, comparing both sides.
✔ **Examine for any obvious deformities**
  ▪ Look for a deformity of the clavicle suggesting an old fracture, a prominent sternoclavicular joint suggesting previous trauma and subluxation at the joint, or prominence of the acromioclavicular joint (also suggesting subluxation or OA).
✔ **Look for muscle wasting**
  ▪ Look particularly at the deltoid, which encases the head of the humerus; this may suggest disuse atrophy, possibly related to pain or damage to the axillary nerve with its characteristic loss of sensation in the regimental badge area (the lateral aspect of the shoulder).
✔ **Check for symmetry**
  ▪ Look at the neck creases, supraclavicular fossa and scapulae for asymmetry in shape, site and size.
  ▪ Look for winging of the scapula. This occurs as a result of damage to the long thoracic nerve, leading to paralysis of the serratus anterior muscle.
✔ **Examine for scars and swelling**

Feel
✔ **Check the temperature**
✔ **Check for tenderness**
  ▪ Feel over both the bony structures and the soft tissues in a systematic fashion.
  ▪ Don't forget to palpate in the axilla for the humeral head.
  ▪ Is the tenderness widespread or localised at the joint?
    – Localised tenderness is seen in adhesive capsulitis, tears of the rotator cuff, tumours, infections, arthritis, subluxations and exostoses.
    – Diffuse tenderness is seen in infection and calcifying supraspinatus tendinitis.
  ▪ Palpate the long head of the biceps tendon for tenderness.

Move
Assess active and passive shoulder movements in the different planes of action. Remember to feel for crepitations on passive movements.
✔ **Check abduction (0–170°)**
  ▪ Observe whilst the patient actively abducts both arms, and look from the front and back. In the absence of any significant pathology, this full range of movement will be pain free and easy for the patient to do.
  ▪ If the patient has difficulty in initiating active abduction, this suggests pathology of the rotator cuff, most likely a tear. If the patient cannot do this at all, you can

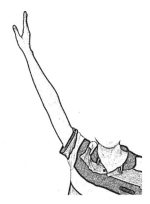

Figure 10.12: Shoulder abduction

> take the arm for him or her and attempt to passively move it, thereby illustrating integrity of the glenohumeral joint. Once fully abducted, ask the patient to keep the arm there, illustrating integrity of the deltoid muscle.
>
> ■ If the patient cannot actively abduct the shoulder and you cannot passively do this, next isolate the scapula and abduct the arm using your other hand, if this is not possible, then a fixed glenohumeral joint is present.
>
> ■ **The painful arc:**
>   – If pain occurs between 60° and 120° of movement, this implicates subacromial impingement of the rotator cuff.
>   – If pain is present between 120° and 180°, this indicates acromioclavicular impingement of the rotator cuff or OA of this joint.

✔ **Check adduction (50°):** Keep the shoulder still, flex at the elbow and move across the chest to the opposite shoulder.

✔ **Check forward flexion (0–165°):** Lift the arm forwards until it is straight up.

✔ **Check backward extension (0–60°):** Swing the arm directly backwards.

✔ **External rotation (70°)**

> ■ Flex the elbow to 90° and adduct to the side of the lateral chest wall, then rotate outwards.
>
> ■ Rotation is reduced in adhesive capsulitis and increased in a tear of the subscapularis muscle.

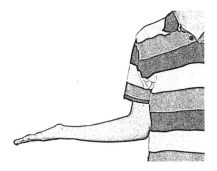

Figure 10.13: External rotation

✔ **Internal rotation**
- Ask the patient to touch the opposite scapula with the dorsum of his or her hand.
- Again, this cannot be done in adhesive capsulitis.

Special tests

It is acceptable to do a mini neurological examination to assess muscle power, as many shoulder pathologies present clinically with muscle weakness.

✔ **Check serratus anterior**

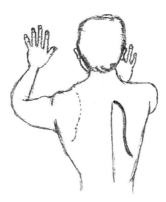

Figure 10.14: Winged scapula

- Perform the **wall test**.
- The patient is asked to push against a wall; this may demonstrate a winged scapula.

This test can also be done during inspection when checking for asymmetry of the scapulae.

✔ **Check deltoid**
- To test this, the patient abducts his or her shoulder against resistance from the examining hand.
- You may wish to test sensation over the regimental badge area.
- Decreased sensation and power may be due to an axillary nerve palsy.

✔ **Check rotator cuff muscles**

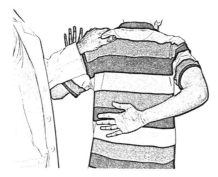

Figure 10.15: Gerber's lift-off test

- **Subscapularis:** To conduct Gerber's lift-off test, with the shoulder in internal rotation on the patient's back, ask the patient to lift his or her hand off against resistance.
- **Infraspinatus:** This uses external rotation against resistance.

You are looking for weakness and/or pain, which suggest cuff tears and tendinitis, respectively.

Rotator cuff impingement can be tested for via the various eponymously named impingement tests. As a positive result is indicated by pain, we suggest you avoid these tests. The most popular method is the Neer impingement test, where a positive result is demonstrated when the shoulder is maximally forward flexed and internally rotated, which will cause the greater tuberosity to 'impinge' against the anterior and inferior surface of the acromion, leading to pain.

✔ **Check biceps tendon**
- Sometimes referred to as the **Popeye test**, a ruptured long head of biceps will bulge prominently when the elbow is flexed against resistance.

The below-mentioned tests are of quite an advanced level and should be offered to an examiner depending on the case. Most examiners would be happy that you are simply aware they exist.

✔ **Perform anterior and posterior drawer tests**

These tests check for anterior and posterior dislocation, respectively.
- **Anterior drawer test:** With the patient lying supine, hold the relaxed arm in one hand and abduct the shoulder to 90°. Flex and externally rotate the shoulder only slightly. With your free hand, stabilise the scapula with your thumb on the coracoid process and the rest of your fingers behind. Now try and pull the humeral head anteriorly. You are looking for apprehension from the patient and clicks or actual anterior movement, all suggestive of anterior dislocation.
- **Posterior drawer test:** With the patient lying supine, abduct his or her shoulder to 90° and keep in slight flexion, with the elbow also flexed. With your other hand, place your thumb just lateral to the coracoid and push the humeral head backwards whilst simultaneously internally rotating the shoulder and flexing it to 80°. In a posterior dislocation, you will feel backward displacement.

The apprehension and relocation tests are modifications of the above tests and are used to assess a patient for chronic anterior instability.

Complete the examination
✔ **Further examination**
- *'To complete my examination, I would like to perform a complete neurological and vascular examination of the upper limbs, as well as examine the neck and elbow'.*
- If you felt there was pathology, you can ask to see the X-rays at this point; if not, then offer to look at them when presenting your findings.

It is also important to examine the cervical spine, as shoulder weakness and pain can be due to neck pathology.

✔ Thank the patient
✔ Wash your hands
✔ Present your findings

Viva questions

Q1 Which muscles make up the rotator cuff?
 ▪ Supraspinatus, Infraspinatus, Teres minor and Subscapularis.

A commonly used mnemonic is **SITS**.

Q2 What is the aetiology of a winged scapula?
 ▪ This is essentially a long thoracic nerve palsy leading to a weak serratus anterior muscle.
 ▪ Damage to the long thoracic nerve can occur during axillary surgery, e.g. a radical mastectomy with axillary node clearance.

(Average Response)

 ▪ It can be damaged secondary to a brachial plexus injury or viral infection of C5, 6 and 7.
 ▪ Rare causes include muscular dystrophies; it is therefore important to perform a careful neurological examination of the upper limbs.

(Good Response)

A winged scapula is usually managed conservatively in cases of minimal disability. Operative repair involves tendon transfer to stabilise the scapula.

10.6 HANDS

Most cases you will see in finals consist of spot diagnoses, although any examiner asking you to 'look at these hands' will still expect you to do a cursory examination focusing specifically on features suggestive of your initial diagnosis. Therefore, we have taken this same approach with the common cases you are likely to encounter if presented with a patient's hands to examine.

Authors' Top Tip

It is also worth pointing out that if you see a pillow, as will often be the case, offer it to the patient so that he or she may rest the hands comfortably on it as you perform your examination.

Case 1: Rheumatoid arthritis hands

Instructions: Please perform a focused examination of this woman's hands.

Key features to look for:
Look
 ▪ **Symmetry:** Symmetrical involvement (look at both hands).

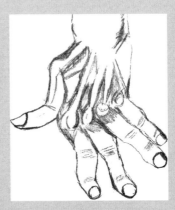

Figure 10.16: Rheumatoid hands

- **Characteristic deforming features:** Ulnar deviation, Z thumb, boutonnières and swan neck deformities.
- **Swellings:** Particularly at the MCPJ and PIPJ; with characteristic sparing of the DIPJ.
- **Nails:** Signs of psoriasis (pitting).
- **Muscle wasting:** Particularly of the dorsal interossei (especially the first web space).
- **Elbows:** Psoriatic plaques or rheumatoid nodules.
- **Behind the ears:** Psoriatic plaques.

Feel
Palpate over any swollen joints, checking for:
- **Temperature and tenderness:** Seen in active RA.
- **Elbows:** Palpate for subcutaneous nodules.

Move
- **Motor function assessment:** Wrist flexion/extension, finger apposition and power grip.
- **Sensation:** Median nerve entrapment leading to carpal tunnel syndrome; the ulnar nerve may be affected due to rheumatoid nodules at the elbow.

Authors' Top Tip

Don't forget that patients with RA have tender joints, so always ask the patient about pain before moving any part of his or her body.

Complete the exam
Present your findings:
- *'This patient appears to have signs suggestive of RA; can I see the X-rays please?'*

(Average Response)

- *'This patient has a symmetrical deforming polyarthropathy. I would like to examine for extra-articular features of RA. May I see the X-rays?'*

  (Good Response)

- *'This patient has a symmetrical deforming polyarthropathy. I would like to examine for extra-articular features of RA, assess the patient's functional status and check to see if the RA is active or quiescent. May I see the X-rays please?'*

  (Honours Response)

You should be aware of the extra-articular features of RA and the five common causes of anaemia in RA (although these are commonly asked for in medical finals). You can then proceed by discussing the X-ray features of RA versus OA, in addition to discussing whether you think the patient has active or quiescent arthritis. It is also worth addressing the patient's functional status, e.g. by asking the patient to unbutton part of his or her shirt.

Remember, management will involve a MDT approach with input from the OT and physiotherapists, as well as the GP and rheumatologist for consideration of specialist disease modifying anti-rheumatic drugs (DMARDs).

The main differential diagnosis will be psoriatic arthropathy, which is likely if there are signs of psoriasis and the articular changes are asymmetrical.

Case 2: Boutonnière deformity

Instructions: Please examine this woman's hands and give me a spot diagnosis.

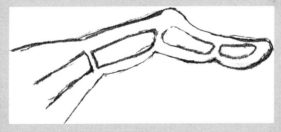

Figure 10.17: Boutonnière deformity

Key features to look for:
- Flexion of the PIPJ with hyperextension of the DIPJ.
- This is usually seen as an additional feature in a patient with rheumatoid hands.

Complete the exam

Case 3: Osteoarthritis of the hands

Instructions: Please examine this woman's hands and give me a spot diagnosis.

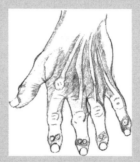

Figure 10.18: OA hands

Key features to look for:
- Heberden's nodes at the distal phalanx; Bouchard's nodes at the PIPJ.

<u>Complete the examination</u>
Some patients may have features of both RA and OA, i.e. a mixed picture; if so, examine as above for RA. OA of the hands is generally a non-deforming polyarthropathy compared to RA hands.

Case 4: Trigger finger (stenosing tenosynovitis)

Instructions: Please examine this woman's hands and give me a spot diagnosis.

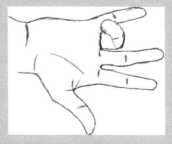

Figure 10.19: Trigger finger

Key features to look for:
- At least one finger is stuck in flexion while the others are straightened.
- On forced extension, the finger subsequently straightens with an audible click.
- Palpate for a nodule over the tendon sheath just proximal to the affected finger; this may be tender.

<u>Complete the examination</u>

Viva questions

Q1 What are the causes of trigger finger?

(Difficult Question)

- Thickening of the flexor tendon sheath as it enters the digit.
- This can be caused by trauma, but it is generally idiopathic. There is an association with rheumatoid arthritis.

Operative repair involves incising the sheath to release the tendon. Some patients benefit from steroid injections.

Case 5: Dupuytren's contracture

Instructions: Please perform a focused examination of this man's hands.

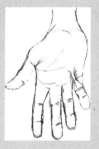

Figure 10.20: Dupuytren's contracture

Key features to look for:
- Thickened, nodular hypertrophy of the palmar aponeurosis may be visible with a fixed-flexion deformity of the little and ring fingers (at the PIPJ and MCPJ).
- You may see a Z-plasty scar (indicating previous surgery).
- It will be painless on palpation; you will feel a thickened nodule fixed to the skin.

Complete the exam
Offer to assess the other hand and assess the feet for similar contractures.

(Good Response)

Offer to assess for the presence of a Dupuytren's diathesis by examining the feet for Ledderhose's disease and the MCPJ for Garrod's pads, plus asking about a family history and, specifically in the male patient, the presence of Peyronie's disease.

(Honours Response)

Examiner's Anecdote

'The fact he even knew about the Dupuytren's diathesis was enough for me. He scored higher than any of the other candidates I have seen today'.

Viva questions

Q1   What are the causes of Dupuytren's contracture?

(Difficult Question)

- It is idiopathic and can be familial.
- Other causes are thought to be related to trauma (especially manual labour), alcohol consumption, epilepsy and consequently anti-epileptics (phenytoin).
- Diabetes .
- Dupuytren's diathesis.

Diathesis is a term that generally means a greater tendency towards a condition. In the case of Dupuytren's, a Dupuytren's diathesis is essentially a more aggressive form of Dupuytren's, specifically where such patients also have other coexisting connective tissue disorders such as Ledderhose's disease (plantar fibromatosis), Peyronie's disease (affecting penile curvature) and the presence of Garrod's nodes on the knuckle pads, amongst others.

Authors' Top Tip

However, do not offer Peyronie's disease as one of the first causes you mention, as this is quite rare. In particular, do not embarrass yourself by offering this diagnosis if the patient is a lady!

Q2   What are your differentials?

(Difficult Question)

- The same as for any contracted hand, which would include:
  - Ulnar nerve palsy.
  - Klumpke's palsy.
  - Volkmann's ischaemic contracture and contractures due to burns.

10.7   BACK

This examination came up during one of the author's final-year OSCEs, so be prepared. Cases that could potentially come up include scoliosis, ankylosing spondylitis and lumbar disc herniation.

Clinical examination

Introduction
As for any clinical encounter (*see* Chapter 1, Principles of a clinical encounter).

Look
✔ **Observe the patient from the front**
- Facing the patient, observe the chest wall for any *pectus excavatum* or *carinatum*.
- Look at the level of the shoulders and hips for asymmetry.

✔ **Observe the patient from the side**
- Look for the normal spinal curvature, e.g. *'I can see the patient has a normal cervical lordosis, an adequate thoracic kyphosis and a normal lumbar lordosis'.*

Table 10.3: Kyphosis and lordosis of the spine

Spine	Finding	Pathology
Cervical	**Increased lordosis**	Ankylosing spondylitis
	Loss of lordosis (flexion deformity)	RA
Thoracic	**Increased kyphosis**	TB (gibbus deformity); wedge fracture of a vertebral body due to osteoporosis or metastatic carcinoma; Scheuermann's osteochondritis; ankylosing spondylitis
	Kyphoscoliosis	Scoliosis
Lumbar	**Loss of lordosis**	Ankylosing spondylitis; disc prolapse; OA; old age
	Increased lordosis	Normal variant, secondary to fixed flexion deformity at the hip

✔ **Observe the patient from the back**
- **Scars:** Surgical scars from spinal operations.
- **Skin changes**, e.g. café au lait spots (neurofibromatosis) or hairy patches (spina bifida).
- **Spinal deviation:** Any lateral curvatures or obvious scoliosis.

✔ **Screen for scoliosis**
- Run your fingers down the spine and look for any lateral curvatures.
- Perform the forward flexion test (Adam's Test):
  - Ask the patient to fold his or her hands together with the elbows extended (this moves the scapula out the way); the patient should then bend forward as far as possible.
  - You will see a rib hump or prominence, suggesting a true structural scoliosis.

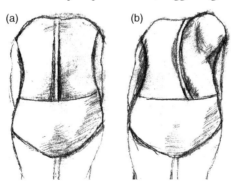

(a)   (b)

Figure 10.21: Scoliosis test *(a: normal test, b: positive test)*

✔ **Examine the gait (*see* Section 10.1)**
✔ **Perform the wall test**
- When the patient stands with his or her back against a wall, this can accentuate any spinal deformity.
- Normally, patients should be able to touch the wall with the heels, buttocks, scapula and occiput simultaneously.

Feel
✔ **Palpate for tenderness**
  ▪ **Spinous processes:** Gently palpate from the occiput to the sacrum and around the sacroiliac joint; feel for any obvious steps (spondylolisthesis).
  ▪ **Paravertebral area:** Palpate the muscles around the spinal column.
  ▪ **Percussion of the spine:** From the occiput to the sacrum.

Tenderness may be due to a prolapsed intervertebral disc, a pathological fracture or deep-seated infections such as TB or *staph aureus* sepsis.

Move
Cervical spine:
✔ **Check forward flexion (80°)**
  ▪ Ask the patient to place his or her chin on the chest.
✔ **Check extension (50°)**
  ▪ Ask the patient to look up at the ceiling and lean the head back as far as possible.
✔ **Check lateral flexion (45°)**
  ▪ Ask the patient to touch his or her ear to the shoulder, repeating on the opposite side.
✔ **Check rotation (80°)**
  ▪ Ask the patient to look over his or her shoulder, repeating on the opposite side.

Thoracic and lumbar spine:
✔ **Check rotation (40°)**
  ▪ With the patient seated, ask him or her to place the arms across the chest, and while keeping their hips still, twist the body to the left and right.
✔ **Check forward flexion (thoracic 45°, lumbar 60°)**
  ▪ With the patient standing, ask him or her to bend forward as far as possible, keeping the knees straight whilst trying to touch the toes.
  ▪ If this is limited, consider performing Schober's test *(see below)*.
✔ **Check extension (30°)**
  ▪ With the patient standing, ask him or her to place the hands on the hips and lean back as far as possible. If this is painful, consider a prolapsed disc.
✔ **Check lateral flexion (30°)**
  ▪ With the patient standing, ask him or her to move the hands down the sides of the leg, leaning as far as possible and repeating on the opposite side.

Special tests
✔ **Schober's test**
  ▪ This assesses whether a limited forward flexion is lumbar or thoracic in origin.
  ▪ **Lumbar spine:** With the patient standing, find the dimples of Venus to act as a reference point. Using a tape measure, mark a point 10 cm above this reference point (Point A), then mark another point 5 cm (halfway) above this reference point (Point B). Measure the distance between point A and B with the patient in maximal forward flexion; normally there should be an increase of up to 10 cm

between the two points. If there is a minimal increase of <3 cm, this suggests restriction in the lumbar spine.

- **Thoracic spine:** With the patient standing, find the prominent T1 vertebra and use this as a reference point. Using a tape measure, mark a point 20 cm below the reference point. With the patient in maximal forward flexion, measure the distance between the two points; normally, there should be an increase of up to 8 cm. A minimal increase suggests a restriction of the thoracic spine.

✔ **Provocation tests**

These tests are positive if the patient experiences pain, so warn the patient appropriately.

- **Straight-leg raise:** With the patient supine, keeping the knee fully extended, straight-leg raise to assess the sciatic nerve; again, the test is positive if pain is felt. Dorsiflexing the foot will aggravate any pain further (the sciatic stretch). Repeat on the opposite side. Crossing the normal leg over whilst straight-leg raising the other leg may produce pain on the affected side; this suggests a prolapsed lumbar disc.

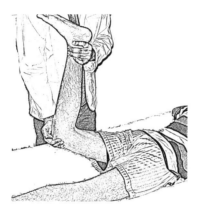

Figure 10.22: Femoral stretch test

- **Femoral nerve (L2, 3, 4) stretch test:** With the patient prone, flex the knee as far as possible and then extend the hip by lifting the knee off the examining bed. Pain is seen in high lumbar lesions. Repeat on the opposite side.

Complete the examination

✔ **Further examination**
- '*To complete my examination, I would like to perform a complete neurological and vascular examination of the upper and lower limbs. In addition, I would like to examine the hip and abdomen*'.
- If you feel there is pathology, you can ask to see the X-rays at this point; if not, then offer to look at them when presenting your findings.

✔ **Thank the patient**

✔ **Wash your hands**

✔ **Present your findings**

An ESR may be a useful screening test to looking for more significant pathology, ranging from malignancy to TB. In clinical practice, when confronted with back pain, ensure you examine the abdomen screening for AAA and organomegaly due to malignancy (particularly a pelvic mass). You must also perform a DRE, checking for signs of prostate carcinoma and documenting anal tone plus the preservation of perineal sensation. You should also examine the hips for OA, which may be the cause of pain. Although more common in medical finals, it would be useful to be aware of the 'red flag' signs of back pain in case you are questioned:

Table 10.4: Red flag signs/symptoms

Variable	Red flag sign/symptom
Age	<20 years or >55 years.
Onset	Acute onset in an elderly patient.
Site	Thoracic pain.
Pattern of pain	▪ Pain increases on lying supine. ▪ Constant or progressive pain. ▪ Morning stiffness. ▪ Nocturnal pain. ▪ Leg claudication (seen in spinal stenosis).
Alarm symptoms	Fever, night sweats, weight loss.
Medical history	Known history of malignancy; immunosuppressed patient, e.g. HIV-positive; on steroids; diabetic; recent infection.
Examination findings	▪ Abdominal/pelvic mass. ▪ Neurological disturbance: loss of perineal sensation. ▪ Sphincter disturbance (altered bladder or bowel function).

Viva questions

Q1 What are the typical X-ray appearances of ankylosing spondylitis?
  - ▪ The so-called 'bamboo' spine appearance on an AP view (this is due to ossification of the intervertebral discs)

Clinically, patients demonstrate the 'question mark' sign, when the body resembles the figure of a question mark due to a fixed kyphosis with compensating cervical spine extension and a loss of the normal lumbar lordosis. Patients have a stiff spine and complain of back pain. There is an association with inflammatory bowel disease and Reiter's syndrome, etc. Patients have a raised ESR and most are human leukocyte antigen (HLA) B27 positive.

Q2 Do you know of any types of scoliosis?

(Honours Question)

  - ▪ Scoliosis can be compensatory, postural, or truly structural.
  - ▪ Compensatory scoliosis is seen in those with true leg shortening.
  - ▪ Postural scoliosis is commonly seen in young girls and is self-limiting.
  - ▪ A truly structural scoliosis occurs when the vertebrae are actually deformed; this is commonly idiopathic, but conditions such as spina bifida and polio are known causes.

10.8 FRACTURES

A fracture is a break in the continuity of bone, complicated by a soft tissue injury.

(Surgical Definition)

The majority of fractures you will see in your clinical practice will occur as a result of trauma. Significant blood loss can occur from a fractured pelvis or long bone; patients therefore need to be resuscitated as the first step in their management. So whenever you are asked about fracture management, always follow ATLS guidelines with the initial aim of resuscitating the patient, then imaging and reducing the deformity with subsequent immobilization and later rehabilitation.

Open fractures generally require broad-spectrum antibiotics, typically benzylpenicillin (due to the risk of *Clostridium perfringens* infection), tetanus prophylaxis (if appropriate) and operative management for irrigation, plus debridement and usually open reduction and internal fixation (ORIF). These patients are therefore classified as orthopaedic emergencies. More ambitious students may wish to have an understanding of the healing process involved in bone repair and modelling. The general complications of fractures are commonly discussed in finals.

Describing fractures on X-rays

Whenever you are presented with a plain film skeletal radiograph, always begin with the general principles of image reporting *(see Chapter 12)*. Specifically for orthopaedic X-rays, you need to address the following points:

General features
✔ **Check patient details**
  ▪ Always check patient details. Often the patient's details and the date of the film have been anonymised for finals, and as a result, some candidates feel this excuses them from checking those details. Do not be fooled – make it a habit to check patient details, as not doing so in the exams promotes bad clinical practice. In addition, there is usually a mark on the score sheet for checking patient details, so you will lose out on easy marks if you neglect checking this.
  ▪ Even if you do not know the patient's details, it is acceptable to either state that you would check, or as *we* recommend, anonymise your response, e.g. *'This is an X-ray of Patient X, taken on X date'.* This helps the flow of your answer and saves you precious time reading the blacked-out patient details sticker.
✔ **Orientate to body region**
  ▪ Which joint or bone are you looking at, and is it the left or right? (Often this is labelled.)

Authors' Top Tip

Look at some long-bone radiographs before you attend finals, as you do not want to confuse the femur with the humerus. We have seen countless students do so in the past!

  ▪ Use correct anatomical terms.

Examiner's Anecdote

'I could not believe it when he said this was the "leg bone". It was painful trying to get a name out of him. Not knowing the name of common bones at this stage is simply not acceptable'.

✔ **Comment on the adequacy of the film**
- ■ You should accept two views (usually AP and lateral, or any that are 90° to each other).
- ■ If you are only given one view, ask to see the corresponding view. This is important, as a fracture or dislocation may not be visible on an AP film but may become obvious on the lateral.
- ■ You must also be able to see the joint above and the joint below. This is important, especially in a trauma case, as the joint nearby may be fractured or dislocated. This also allows you to comment on axial rotation.

Authors' Top Tip

A common trick used by examiners in finals is to give you a single view only. Turn to the examiner and politely request to see another view before you comment on the first. This demonstrates your understanding of the above principles.

Fracture

✔ **Describe the fracture**
- ■ Site: Where is the fracture? Is it in the distal segment or in the mid-shaft?

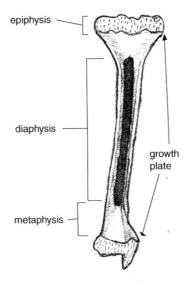

Figure 10.23: Anatomical long bone divisions

- – A long bone is divided into the following anatomical divisions: the epiphysis, the epiphyseal plate, the shaft/diaphysis and the metaphysis (located between the shaft and the epiphyseal plate).

- An accurate description of the site of the fracture is important, as this helps predict healing potential.
- You can also describe the site using anatomical landmarks, e.g. fracture of the neck of femur.
- Often it is easier to describe the location of a fracture of a long bone if you divide the bone into segments, e.g. proximal third, middle third or distal third.
- **Extent:** Complete or incomplete.
- **Pattern:** Transverse, oblique or spiral.
- **Fragments:** Two or more pieces; multiple fragments (comminuted).
✔ **Describe the two ends of the bone (at the fracture site)**
- **Impaction:** Compression of the two ends against each other.
- **Displacement:** Note whether the ends of the bones in the fracture have moved relative to each other; if they have, consider the following:
  - **Extent:** Partial or complete displacement.
  - **Direction:** E.g. dorsal.
  - **Degree of tilt:** Estimate the angle that the distal end of the distal fragment makes relative to its normal anatomical position.

If there is no displacement of bone segments within a fracture, then it is described as still being in its anatomical position.

Special features
✔ **Look for associated injuries**
- **Foreign bodies:** Contamination, e.g. glass, suggesting an open fracture.
- **Soft tissue injuries:** Look for evidence of infection (air from Clostridium infection); swelling.
- **Dislocations:** Fractures in one region may cause dislocation in another, e.g. Monteggia; hence the importance of viewing films of the joint above and below.

Completion
✔ **Present your findings**
- If you are aware of the classification system for the fracture you have been given, then use it, as this will impress the examiner.

Authors' Top Tip

It is not usually obvious from an X-ray if a fracture is open, so it is best to avoid stating if the fracture is open or closed in your presentation.

By far, you are more likely to be presented with an X-ray of a Colles' or neck of femur (NOF) fracture in finals. If, however, you are given an X-ray of a fracture that you are unfamiliar with, do not panic. Following a systematic approach is far more important than recognising the eponymously named fracture at this stage in your career. For completion, we include several other possible fractures that you may come across:

Table 10.5: Miscellaneous fractures

Fracture	Mechanism	Radiological features
Smith's	Sustained through a fall onto a flexed wrist.	The distal radial fracture fragment is displaced volarly (ventrally).
Monteggia	This is a fracture of the proximal third of the ulna, with dislocation of the head of radius that is sustained by either: 1 A fall on an outstretched hand with the forearm in excessive pronation (hyper-pronation injury). 2 A direct blow on the back of the upper forearm.	Classified into four types (dependent upon displacement of the radial head): I – Extension type (60%): Ulna shaft angulates anteriorly (extends), and radial head dislocates anteriorly. II – Flexion type (15%): Ulna shaft angulates posteriorly (flexes), and radial head dislocates posteriorly. III – Lateral type (20%): Ulna shaft angulates laterally (bent to outside), and radial head dislocates to the side. IV – Combined type (5%): Ulna shaft and radial shaft are both fractured and radial head is dislocated, typically anteriorly.
Galeazzi	The Galeazzi fracture is thought to occur after a fall resulting in an axial load on a hyperpronated forearm.	This is a fracture of the radius with dislocation of the distal radio-ulnar joint. It classically involves an isolated fracture of the junction of the distal third and middle third of the radius with associated subluxation or dislocation of the distal radio-ulnar joint.
Scaphoid	This occurs after a fall on an outstretched hand.	Not initially apparent on plain radiographs. Those with tenderness over the scaphoid are put into a cast, and a second set of plain films will be taken 10-12 days later.
Femoral shaft	This is usually the result of a twisting fall when the foot is anchored. It could happen due to direct force (e.g. a motorcycle accident) or due to a pathological fracture (e.g. Paget's).	The fracture is generally in the middle of the shaft. Remember, it is important to exclude an associated pelvic fracture, so do not forget to X-ray the pelvis.
Humerus	Transverse fractures may result from direct trauma to the humerus or a fall on the elbow with an abducted arm. Spiral fractures may result from twisting of the humerus during a fall on the hand. Comminuted fractures usually occur as a result of direct injury; pathological fractures from primary bone tumours, metastatic deposits and osteoporosis.	Fracture of the humeral shaft. Eighty per cent of proximal humerus fractures are non-displaced or minimally displaced.

Case 1: Colles' fracture

Instructions: This man fell on his outstretched hand. Comment on his X-rays.

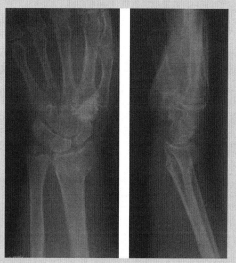

Figure 10.24: Colles' fracture (AP and lateral views)

Key features to note:

- *'These are AP and lateral views of the right wrist of Patient X, taken on X Date.*
- *The most obvious abnormality is that of an incomplete fracture of the distal radius with dorsal displacement of the distal end of the distal fragment on the lateral view'.*

(Average Response)

- *'I cannot see an associated fracture of the ulnar styloid, and there is no obvious impaction or radial shortening'.*

(Good Response)

Completion

- *'In summary, there is a fracture of the distal radius within 2.5 cm of the wrist joint. There is dorsal tilt of the distal fragment, but no associated ulnar styloid fracture.*
- *This is a Colles' Fracture.*
- *I would like to assess the need for reduction by estimating the degree of tilt.*
- *There is >15° dorsal tilt of the distal fragment relative to the radial shaft, therefore an indication for reduction. It may be done under sedation or anaesthesia.*
- *To complete my assessment, I would like to take a look at X-rays of the joint above and the joint below'.*

(Honours Response)

A Colles' is a fracture of the radius within 2.5 cm of the wrist. Classically, this type of fracture is seen following a fall onto an extended, outstretched hand. Clinically, the patient has the so-called 'dinner fork' deformity of the wrist. Be aware that there is an associated fracture of the ulnar styloid process in more than 60% of cases. Other typical radiological features include loss of radial inclination, ulnar angulation of the wrist and impaction with various degrees of comminution of the fractured segment.

If undisplaced, a dorsal splint is applied, and the patient is reviewed in fracture clinic. If slightly displaced, the fracture may be reduced in the Emergency Department using Entonox gas as analgesia for the patient. If grossly displaced, the patient requires reduction under anaesthesia and repeat X-ray to check if the procedure has been successful. Several regional anaesthetic methods are used for this purpose, such as a Bier's or haematoma block.

Viva questions

Q1 What are the complications of this fracture?

(Difficult Question)

Complications of fractures can be divided into general complications seen in any fracture or complications specific to a Colles' fracture.

General complications of any fracture:

- **Immediate:** Damage to the surrounding structures, e.g. bladder injuries in pelvic fractures; nerve and vascular injuries.
- **Early:** Compartment syndrome, haemarthrosis, infection, gas gangrene.
- **Late:** Delayed union, non-union, malunion, avascular necrosis, joint instability, OA. Some patients develop complex regional pain syndrome. Growth disturbance is possible in children.
- **Soft tissue injury complications:** Fat embolism, rhabdomyolysis, stiffness, muscle contractures, nerve compression or entrapment, tendon rupture.

There are other indirect general complications related to the prolonged immobility in many patients. This can range from bedsores to DVT and PEs. Many elderly patients typically develop chest and urinary tract infections whilst as hospital inpatients.

Complications specific to Colles':

- **Malunion:** This is common.
- **Nerve injury:** Including median nerve compression; carpal tunnel syndrome.
- **Joint stiffness:** Stiff upper limb.
- **Tendon rupture:** Of the extensor pollicis longus tendon, several weeks after initial injury.
- **Complex regional pain syndrome.**

Q2 Which bones typically develop avascular necrosis post-injury?
- The scaphoid, the head of femur, the lunate and the body of the talus.

Case 2: Neck of femur fracture

Instructions: This elderly woman fell down the stairs. Comment on her X-rays.

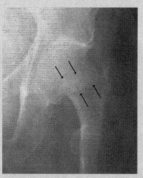

Figure 10.25: Neck of femur fracture

Key features to note:
- *'This is an AP view of the left hip of Patient X, taken on X Date'.*
- **Candidate:** *'I would like to take a look at the lateral view, please'.* **Examiner:** *'Not available. Please continue'.*

Authors' Top Tip

Remember, there will be a mark for checking the second view, so always ask for one, even if it is not available!

- *'The most obvious abnormality is that of an incomplete intracapsular fracture of the neck of femur; it is non-displaced but impacted.*
- *This is a Garden grade I intracapsular fracture.*
- *Coincidentally, I can also see osteoarthritic changes of the hip'.*

Completion
- *'In summary, there is a Garden grade I intracapsular fracture of the left neck of femur.*
- *This is an orthopaedic emergency (see Viva Q2 below).*
- *To complete my assessment, I would like to take a look at X-rays of the joint above and the joint below, as well as a lateral view of the left hip'.*

Viva questions

Q1 How do you classify neck of femur fractures?

(Difficult Question)

Broadly classified into intra- or extracapsular; intracapsular fractures are commonly classified using the Garden classification system:
- **Garden grade I:** Incomplete fracture, impacted, undisplaced.

- **Garden grade II:** Complete fracture with no displacement.
- **Garden grade III:** Complete fracture with partial displacement.
- **Garden grade IV:** Complete fracture, totally displaced.

Remember, the femoral head is at risk of avascular necrosis due to disruption of the retinacular blood supply, so accurate classification is important; this guides operative treatment. Extracapsular fractures tend to be treated with open reduction internal fixation (ORIF) using a dynamic hip screw. Intracapsular Garden grades III and IV usually require femoral head excision and hemiarthroplasty. Grades I and II may be amenable to screws.

Q2 How would you manage this patient?
- *'This is a surgical emergency; I would resuscitate the patient according to ATLS guidelines, ensuring the patient's Airway is patent with C-spine immobilisation in place. I would then assess the patient's Breathing and address Circulation, beginning by inserting two large-bore cannulae into each antecubital fossa whilst taking bloods for further investigations at the same time.*
- *I would also inform my senior at the earliest opportunity'.*

At this point, the examiner will often direct you to the fracture rather than continuing on to managing the trauma call.
- *'Bloods I would request include an FBC, U&E and G&S as part of a preoperative assessment, since the patient is likely to require operative treatment.*
- *I would request AP and lateral views of the hip and pelvis; a preoperative CXR and an ECG.*
- *I would then begin the patient on normal replacement fluids and keep her NBM with adequate pain relief whilst awaiting senior review with a view for operative management'.*

(Good Response)

10.9 PERIPHERAL NERVE INJURIES

In finals, examination of peripheral nerves is common, particularly those of the ulnar, median and radial nerve lesions, so ensure you are familiar with their examination and anatomy; these are common viva questions.

You are essentially performing a peripheral upper- and lower-limb neurological examination, so you can follow the general routine you would do in a medical OSCE. However, there is an emphasis on *inspection, assessment of motor power* and *sensation* in the surgical cases of peripheral nerve palsies, and often examiners will focus your examination to the nerve of interest. Do not forget to check both sides and complete your examination by stating that you would examine the other peripheral nerves.

Below, we discuss all the likely nerve injuries you will come across and the key features to note during your neurological examination. Often it will be obvious that this is a nerve palsy, and you may be asked to focus your examination; the key points below will help you do just this.

10.9.1 The axillary nerve

The axillary nerve is also known as the circumflex nerve and originates from the C5–C6 roots, arising as a branch of the posterior cord of the brachial plexus at the level of the axilla. It supplies the deltoid and teres minor muscles and supplies sensation to the shoulder joint and the inferior part of the deltoid, which is known as the 'regimental badge' area. When the axillary nerve splits from the posterior cord of the brachial plexus, it continues as the radial nerve with C5–T1 roots.

Case 1: Axillary nerve lesion

Instructions: This woman is complaining of weakness in her left shoulder. Please examine.

Key features to look for:
Inspection
- **Muscle wasting:** Damage to the nerve will produce wasting of the deltoid muscle, which may appear as a flat shoulder.

Motor power assessment
- Ask the patient to abduct the arm against resistance that you apply, with one hand placed over the deltoid, feeling for muscular contractions and the second hand at the distal humerus, applying resistance.

Test sensation
- Assess over the regimental badge region; this is important in cases where movement at the shoulder is too painful.
- Remember, it is important to document in the patient's notes the axillary nerve function in cases of shoulder dislocations.

Complete the exam
Note: This nerve lesion is likely to be seen as part of a shoulder examination in finals.

Viva questions

Q1 What are the causes of an axillary nerve palsy?
- The nerve is most commonly damaged as a result of shoulder dislocation, displaced fractures of the surgical neck of the humerus and from compression of the nerve from crutches in the axilla.

10.9.2 The radial nerve

The radial nerve supplies the triceps brachii muscle and the extrinsic extensor muscles at the wrist and the dorsum of the arm. It supplies cutaneous sensation to the dorsum of the hand (except the little finger and the ulnar half of the ring finger, which are supplied by the ulnar nerve). The radial nerve divides into two: the deep branch, known as the posterior interosseous, and the superficial radial, which supplies the radial side of the dorsum of the hand.

Case 2: Radial nerve lesion

Instructions: This woman is complaining of weakness in her left hand. Please examine her hand.

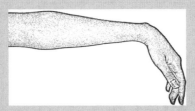

Figure 10.26: Radial nerve lesions

Key features to look for:

Inspection

- **Muscle Wasting:** This refers to wasting of the forearm muscles; wasting in the triceps region would suggest a proximal lesion.
- There may be a wrist drop.

Motor power assessment

- **Assess function of the extensors:** Start with the elbow flexed and the dorsum of the hand facing upwards (in pronation). Isolating just proximally to the wrist, ask the patient to straighten her fingers; next repeat this against resistance offered by your fingers, and finally ask the patient to extend at the wrist joint as you apply resistance to the dorsum of the hand with the dorsum of your hand.

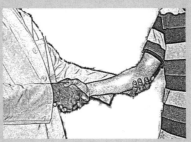

Figure 10.27: Supinator function

- **Assess function of supinator:** With the elbow held in extension to remove the action of the biceps, ask the patient to supinate, then pronate her hand; then repeat this as you apply resistance, which is most easily done by grasping the patient's hand in yours.
- **Assess function of brachioradialis:** This is done by visual inspection and palpation. The patient holds her arm flexed at the elbow and the hand in mid-pronation/supination. The patient is then asked to flex at the elbow whilst you apply resistance, with one hand applied just proximal from the wrist and the fingers of your other hand over the brachioradialis muscle.

- **Assess function of triceps:** The shoulder is held in extension, and the elbow hangs at 45° relative to this; the patient is then asked to extend the elbow and repeat this against resistance offered by you. Ensure movement occurs from the elbow and not the shoulder, as you are assessing the function of the triceps.

Test sensation
- Assess for a sensory disturbance on the dorsum of the hand, most importantly over the anatomical snuffbox (the first dorsal interosseus) and the back of the forehand.

Complete the exam
In a nerve lesion, there will be loss of power and sensation. The site of the lesion can be accurately estimated from the pattern of muscle weakness; for example, triceps weakness suggests a lesion at the mid-humerus, i.e. a high radial nerve lesion. At undergraduate level, you are not expected to localise the site of the lesion from clinical assessment.

Viva questions

Q1 What are the causes of a radial nerve palsy?

The radial nerve can be damaged at any point along its anatomical course. Causes of a radial nerve palsy can be divided into damage that occurs as a result of either injury or long-term pressure to the nerve:
- **Injury to the nerve.**
  - Pressure from ill-fitting crutches ('crutch palsy'), from a chair (the so-called 'Saturday night palsy') or pressure on the nerve when the patient is in deep sleep, such as after alcohol intoxication, with the arm hanging over the back of a chair.
  - Fractures of the mid-humerus/Monteggia's.
  - As a complication of surgery in this region.
  - Elbow dislocations.
- **Long-term pressure.**
  - If a tourniquet is applied for a prolonged period or at too high a pressure ('tourniquet palsy').
  - Compression of the nerve caused by localised swelling or injury to adjacent structures.

(Good Response)

Q2 What further tests do you think this patient should have?

(Difficult Question)

- Further tests may include plain radiographs assessing for fractures.
- MRI of the head, neck and shoulder.
- EMG and nerve conduction tests.

10.9.3 The ulnar nerve

The ulnar nerve descends from the medial cord of the brachial plexus with roots derived from C8-T1. It is a very superficial nerve that is neither protected by muscles or bone, making it the largest unprotected nerve in the body. It descends on the posterior surface of the humerus, travelling behind the medial epicondyle and the cubital tunnel, entering the forearm between the heads of flexor carpi ulnaris; after this, it descends with the ulna, ultimately entering the palm of the hand.

The ulnar nerve gives off branches along its course in the forearm and the hand; together they innervate the following:

Table 10.6: Branches of the ulnar nerve in the forearm

Branches	Supplies
Muscular branch	Flexor carpi ulnaris, flexor digitorum profundus (half)
Palmar branch	Supplies cutaneous sensation to the little finger and ulnar half of the ring finger on the palmar surface and the nails
Dorsal branch	Supplies cutaneous sensation to the little finger and ulnar half of the ring finger on the dorsal aspect

Table 10.7: Branches of the ulnar nerve in the hand

Branches	Supplies
Superficial branch	Palmaris brevis
Deep branch	The hypothenar muscles (opponens digiti minimi, abductor digiti minimi, flexor digiti minimi brevis) Adductor pollicis Ulnar third and fourth lumbrical muscles (first radial two lumbricals are supplied by the median nerve) Dorsal and palmar interossei

Case 3: Ulnar nerve lesion

Instructions: This woman is complaining of weakness in her left hand. Please examine her hand.

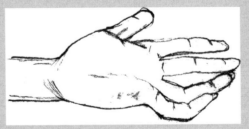

Figure 10.28: Ulnar nerve lesions

Key features to look for:
Inspection
- **Muscle wasting:** In the forearm, this is wasting over the medial side (flexor carpi ulnaris, flexor digitorum profundus). In the hand, the hypothenar eminence and the third and fourth lumbricals may be wasted. Also, look in the first web space, where wasting of the first dorsal interosseous muscle can be seen.
- **Claw hand:** Here, the MCPJs are in extension and the IPJs are in marked flexion, involving the little and ring fingers and occurring due to paralysis of the interossei and lumbricals from a lesion proximal to flexor digitorum profundus. In cases where the MCPJ is flexed, the lesion is distal to the flexor digitorum profundus (FDP).
- **Scars:** Of previous injury anywhere along its course, i.e. at the elbow, wrist or forearm.
- **Skin changes:** Ulceration, trophic changes.

Motor power assessment
- **Assess function of the interossei:** Ask the patient to extend her fingers. Next, ask the patient to grip a sheet of plain paper between the little and ring finger. Now gently try to pull the paper out of the patient's grip, noting how easy this is. If there is paralysis of these muscles, the patient will be unable to grip the paper.
- **Assess function of the first dorsal interosseus:** Whilst inspecting and palpating this muscle, the patient's hand is placed palm down on a table, isolating its function; ask the patient to push the index finger against resistance from your index finger.
- **Assess function of the abductor digiti minimi:** The patient's fingers are extended, and you will use your index finger to force the little finger in adduction while the patient is told to prevent you from doing this; note the resistance offered.

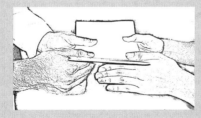

Figure 10.29: Froment's test

- **Assess function of the adductor pollicis (Froment's sign):** Place a sheet of paper between the thumb and index finger; ask the patient to hold onto this whilst you gently pull it away. If the adductor pollicis is paralysed, you will see the patient flexing at the IPJ in order to keep hold of the paper; this is a positive Froment's sign.

- **Assess function of the flexor carpi ulnaris:** Ask the patient to prevent you from extending her flexed wrist, and note the resistance.

Authors' Top Tip

As you will not be allowed to bring paper with you into the examination, paper will be provided for you, so ask for it when performing the above tests as needed.

Test sensation

- Assess sensation over the hypothenar eminence, palmar and dorsal aspect of the little and ulnar half of the ring finger.
- Palpate the ulnar nerve at its anatomical location over the medial epicondyle, then palpate proximally and distally to this; you are assessing for paraesthesiae and tenderness.
- Now assess again at this location by flexing and extending the elbow.
- Repeat this at its anatomical location at the wrist, just lateral to flexor carpi ulnaris.

Complete the exam

Again, you will not be expected to differentiate between a distal and proximal lesion through clinical examination at the undergraduate level.

Viva questions

Q1 What are the causes of an ulnar nerve palsy?
The ulnar nerve can be damaged anywhere along its anatomical course. The most common causes of damage, starting proximally, are:

Table 10.8: Causes of an ulnar nerve palsy

Site	Cause
At the level of the brachial plexus	Tumour (Pancoast's), trauma, cervical rib
Level of the medial epicondyle	Local pressure, friction, trauma or from being stretched (seen in cubitus valgus or OA)
Around the elbow	Supracondylar fractures, dislocations, osteophytic encroachment, golfer's elbow (medial epicondylitis); as a result of compression from the two heads of flexor carpi ulnaris, which may give rise to cubital tunnel syndrome (paraesthesiae brought on when the elbow is in a flexed position)
At the wrist	Trauma, ganglions, fractures, lacerations, ulnar tunnel syndrome (compression of the nerve as it passes between the pisiform and the hook of the hamate)

Q2 Would you expect a more proximal ulnar nerve lesion to have a greater degree of clawing in the hand than a more distal one?

(Honours Question)

- No, this is known as the ulnar paradox.
- For distal lesions at, e.g. the wrist, an ulnar claw deformity is more pronounced than for a more proximal lesion at, e.g. the elbow.
- This is because a more proximal lesion causes weakness in the ulnar half of the FDP, whereas a distal lesion does not.
- In a more proximal lesion, the weakness of the FDP results in a decreased degree of flexion of the distal interphalangeal joints (DIPJs) of the little and ring fingers, which subsequently results in a less pronounced claw deformity.
- As the FDPs are not weak in a distal lesion, the deformity will therefore be greatly exaggerated in comparison.

Authors' Top Tip

This question is commonly used by examiners to catch out candidates, as it tests a candidate's understanding of anatomy. In fact, if you even mentioned the term 'ulnar paradox', most consultants would be impressed that you'd even heard of it.

10.9.4   The median nerve

The median nerve originates from the brachial plexus and is formed by both the medial and lateral cords with roots derived from C5–T1. The median nerve courses down the arm, arising at the cubital fossa; just before this point, it gives off an articular branch to the upper part of the arm. The median nerve gives off branches along its course.

In the forearm it gives off two branches: the anterior interosseous and the palmar cutaneous branch. Here it innervates the anterior compartment of the forearm and all the muscles in it, except the flexor carpi ulnaris and the ulnar half of the FDP, which are both supplied by the ulnar nerve.

The median nerve passes through the carpel tunnel, deep to the flexor retinaculum at the wrist, and is susceptible to compression at this point, which would lead to carpel tunnel syndrome. It gives off a recurrent branch and multiple cutaneous branches in the hand. It gives motor supply to the lateral two lumbricals and the thenar eminence, with the remaining intrinsic muscles of the hand being supplied by the ulnar nerve.

Use the mnemonic '**LOAF**' to recall the muscles in the hand supplied by the median nerve:

L: Lateral two lumbricals.
O: Opponens pollicis.
A: Abductor pollicis brevis.
F: Flexor pollicis brevis.

The median nerve supplies cutaneous sensation to the lateral three-and-a-half fingers on the palmar side, and on the dorsum it supplies the distal phalanx of the thumb, index, middle and radial half of the ring finger.

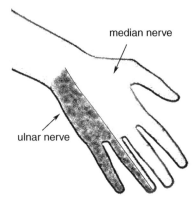

Figure 10.30: Palmar nerve supply

Case 4: Median nerve lesion

Instructions: This woman is complaining of weakness in her left hand. Please examine her hand.

Key features to look for:
Inspection

- **Muscle wasting:** Look at the thenar eminences; in chronic cases, the 'Simian thumb' will become apparent where the thumb lies in the same plane as the palm. There could also be wasting of the lateral aspect of the forearm. Look for the characteristic 'sign of Benediction', where the index finger is kept in extension. (Can be caused by pulp atrophy of the index finger, cigarette burns, i.e. local trauma between the index and middle finger causing denervation.)
- **Scars:** Anywhere along the course of the median nerve, from where it originates at the antecubital fossa.

Motor power assessment

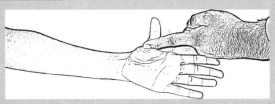

Figure 10.31: Function of the abductor pollicis brevis

- **Assess function of the abductor pollicis brevis:** Place the dorsum of the patient's hand flat on the table so that the palm is facing upwards; ask the patient to lift her thumb off the table; then repeat this, offering resistance.
- **Assess function of the flexor pollicis longus:** Ask the patient to flex the tip of the thumb so there is flexion at the PIPJ; if needed, you can isolate

the thumb by holding just below this joint. If the patient is unable to do this, there is either a lesion of the median nerve itself or of the anterior interosseous branch. To assess function of the latter nerve, ask the patient to bring the tips of the thumb and index finger tightly together. If there is a lesion of the nerve, the tips will be in a position of hyperextension.

- **Assess function of the pronator teres:** With the patient's elbow extended, place one hand over the muscle so you can feel it contracting when it is working, and with your other hand grasp the patient's hand so you can offer resistance; then ask the patient to pronate her hand. In the pronator teres nerve entrapment syndrome, the patient will experience pain on doing this, and there will be muscle tenderness. If the patient is not able to pronate the arm against resistance, this suggests a lesion at or above the elbow.

Test sensation

- Assess sensation over the radial side of the palm and the thumb, index, middle fingers and the thenar eminence.
- Also do this on the dorsum, over the nail beds of the thumb, index and middle fingers.

Special tests

If you suspected nerve compression in the carpel tunnel, you can carry out these additional special tests.

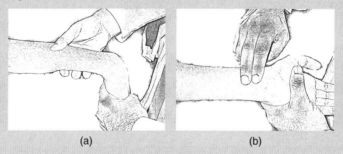

(a)   (b)

Figure 10.32: (a) Phalen's test; (b) Tinel's test

- **Phalen's test:** In this test, the patient is directed to hold both wrists in full flexion for two minutes; it is positive if this reproduces or exacerbates the symptoms.
- **Tinel's test:** Gently tap over the site of the median nerve at the wrist; if this produces paraesthesiae in the median nerve distribution, then consider it to be positive.
- **Tourniquet test:** Inflate a sphygmomanometer cuff for 1–2 minutes to just above the normal systolic pressure, and assess for reproduction of symptoms.
- **Nerve conduction studies:** Although this is not a bed side test, it can also be of benefit, and you should at least offer it when completing your examination.

Complete the examination

Viva questions

Q1 What are the causes of a median nerve palsy?

The median nerve can be damaged anywhere along its course. The most common causes, starting proximally, are:

Table 10.9: Causes of a median nerve palsy

Site	Cause
Cervical nerve root level	Bony spurs, intervertebral discs, tumours
Around the elbow	Dislocations, supracondylar fractures, teres nerve entrapment syndrome (in pronator)
At the forearm	Fractures (anterior interosseous nerve)
At the wrist	Fractures, dislocations, lacerations (including those sustained during suicide attempts), compression of the carpel tunnel (pregnancy, hypothyroidism, acromegaly, multiple myeloma)

Q2 How would you treat a patient with carpal tunnel syndrome?

(Difficult Question)

Conservative measures

- Night-time application of a wrist splint (with the wrist in a neutral position).
- Steroid injection (just proximal to the carpal tunnel).

Surgical measures

- Decompression of the carpal tunnel (can be performed either open or endoscopically).

More ambitious students may wish to learn the borders of the carpal tunnel as this would impress an examiner.

10.9.5   Lower limb nerves

These are less likely to be assessed individually in finals, but still be aware of the features you may wish to look for on clinical examination:

Table 10.10: Proximal lower limb peripheral nerve injuries

Nerve		Features to Remember
Sciatic	**General**	The common peroneal and tibial nerves are derived from the sciatic nerve; they supply muscles of the lower leg (see below). The sciatic nerve can be injured during pelvic surgery, pelvic fractures and posterior dislocations of the hip.
	Examination	**Inspection:** Look for muscle wasting in the distribution of the muscles supplied by the sciatic nerve (hamstrings), tibial nerve (calf), peroneal muscles (superficial peroneal), medial and lateral plantar nerves (muscles of the foot). Observe for foot drop (common peroneal nerve). **Sensation:** Sensory loss on the skin over the hamstrings, over the calf and sole of the foot. **Motor:** Assess for knee and ankle jerk; assess knee flexion and hip extension.

(Continued)

Table 10.10: Proximal lower limb peripheral nerve injuries (*Continued*)

Nerve		Features to Remember
Femoral	**General**	Can be damaged in pelvic fractures, secondary to trauma, or from direct pressure from tumours or a haematoma present in the iliacus muscle. Damage can also occur as a result of iatrogenic injury, e.g. during hip arthroplasty, abdominoplasty or pelvic surgery.
	Examination	**Inspection:** Quadriceps muscle wasting. **Sensation:** Along the distribution of the nerve using a pin prick. **Motor:** Ask the patient to flex the hip while you apply counter traction – here you are assessing the function of the iliopsoas muscle. Next, ask the patient to extend the flexed knee against resistance to assess quadriceps function.

Table 10.11: Distal lower limb peripheral nerve injuries

Nerve		Features to remember
Common peroneal	**General**	Can be damaged as a result of trauma at the fibular neck or fracture of the fibula, pressure from plaster casts, hyperflexion of the knee, iatrogenic injury during surgery to the knee, and (interestingly) sitting with habitually crossed legs.
	Examination	**Inspection:** Muscle wasting anteriorly or laterally over the lower leg. **Sensation:** Assess in the first web space supplied by the deep peroneal, and in the area supplied by the superficial peroneal that is the anterior and lateral areas of the lower leg and over the dorsum of the foot. **Motor:** First, assess gait as you classically get a foot drop with loss of ankle and foot dorsiflexion. Here you will witness a high-stepping gait or the patient dragging the foot along the ground. To assess motor function of the deep branch, ask the patient to dorsiflex against resistance provided by your hand to the dorsum of the foot. To assess the superficial branch, ask the patient to evert the foot against resistance.
Tibial	**General**	Commonly damaged from fractures or injury to the back of the knee; injury to the lower leg including tibial fractures, fracture of the medial malleolus, tight plasters, compartment syndrome of the posterior calf.
	Examination	**Inspection:** Wasting of calf muscles, muscles on the sole of the foot, clawing of the toes. **Sensation:** Assess over the sole of the foot, which is supplied by the medial and lateral plantar branches, and also over the distal phalanges and the nail beds which are also supplied by these nerves. One could also assess sensation of the lateral side of the foot, as this is supplied by the sural nerve, but be careful, as this is also formed from a combination of fibres from the common peroneal nerve. **Motor:** Ask the patient to flex the toes against the resistance provided by your fingers.

CHAPTER 11

Surgical procedures and instruments

11.1 SURGICAL PROCEDURES

Increasingly, surgical procedures are being used as separate OSCE stations in finals. You should be aware of the common procedures that you are likely to be asked to perform during your OSCE, as these same procedures will also form the majority of clinical procedures you will be required to perform during your training as a junior doctor, starting with your FY1 year.

Case 1: Urinary catheterisation

Instructions: Please catheterise this male patient.

<u>Introduction</u>
As for any clinical encounter (*see* Chapter 1, Principles of a clinical encounter). Specifically for this case:
✔ **Wash your hands**
✔ **Maintain aseptic technique:** Remember, this procedure needs to be done under sterile conditions, as you have the potential to introduce infection.
✔ **Expose patient adequately:** Ask the patient to fully undress below the waist.
✔ **Prepare your equipment:**
  ■ Open your catheter pack using aseptic technique; ensure you select a male size catheter (16F); or smaller for a female.
  ■ Ensure you have: lignocaine jelly, a drainage bag, a urinary catheter, a balloon syringe containing 10–20 mL of water (whatever the capacity of the catheter balloon may be; this is normally stated on the port that you use to inflate the balloon), a drape, sterile water in a receiver, gauze and a pair of sterile gloves.
  ■ Place a kidney bowel between the patient's legs; this is to catch the urine.

✔ **Position the patient appropriately:** Have the patient lie supine in bed with his or her legs slightly apart, covered initially by a sheet to maintain modesty until you are ready to proceed.

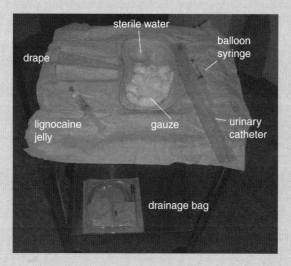

Figure 11.1: Urinary catheterisation pack

Procedure

Ideally you will have an assistant helping you; the examiner will usually offer to do this. But for purposes of the OSCE, assume you are alone.

Now remove the sheet you had used to cover up the patient.

✔ **Put on gloves**
- These should be sterile gloves; put them on using a no-touch technique.

✔ **Clean the genitalia**
- With the fingers of one hand, hold the penis using a sterile swab; this is your clean hand.
- With the other hand, retract the foreskin and clean around the meatus with gauze soaked in sterile water, using concentric circles as you work your way down; this is now your dirty hand.

✔ **Drape the patient**
- Place the penis through the sterile field.

✔ **Apply local anaesthetic**
- Insert generous amounts of lignocaine jelly into the urethra, then gently hold the urethral meatus closed with gauze.
- Say that you would wait for at least 5 minutes for the jelly to take effect before proceeding with catheter insertion.

✔ **Advance the catheter**
- Hold the penis at 90° to the perineum to insert the catheter.

■ Ensure you lubricate the tip of the catheter with some of the lignocaine jelly, which ideally you would have squeezed out onto the sterile field before inserting its entirely into the penis.
■ Insert the catheter slowly and progressively into the urethra, using a no-touch technique.

Authors' Top Tip

Often the catheter is in a sterile sleeve. Use this to aid you, and do not touch the actual catheter as you advance.

✔ **Inflate the balloon**
  ■ When urine flows freely from the end of the catheter into your waiting kidney bowel, you are now in the bladder.
  ■ Inflate the balloon with 10 mL of water in the pre-prepared syringe provided; if it is not pre-prepared, you will obviously need to do this when preparing your equipment.
  ■ If the patient experiences discomfort, stop and reposition the catheter, as the balloon may not be in the bladder.
✔ **Attach the catheter drainage bag**
  ■ Place the bag against the bedside railing.
✔ **Reposition the foreskin**
  ■ This is very important, because if the foreskin is not replaced, the patient will develop a painful paraphimosis.

Completion
✔ **Thank the patient**
✔ **Wash your hands**
✔ **Document the procedure**

Say to the examiner that you would record the residual volume and document the procedure in the patient record, noting the catheter size and volume used to inflate the balloon.

The clinical skills lab is an excellent place to practise this, as the manikins are likely to be very similar to those used in the OSCE.

Authors' Top Tip

When on your clinical placements, always take the initiative and ask to be supervised doing this procedure. Junior doctors will be more than happy to delegate this task to you; this is the best way to learn.

Viva questions

Q1   What are the contraindications of using a urethral catheter?

(Difficult Question)

- It is contraindicated in a polytrauma patient who has suffered a urethral injury. This is usually evident with signs of perineal bruising (in a butterfly distribution) or blood at the urethral meatus.
- It is also contraindicated in any patients known to have urethral strictures, as there is a risk of creating a false passage.

In all cases, say that you would first discuss with a senior for help and advice.

Q2   What would you do if you cannot successfully catheterise the patient?

- Use a larger-sized catheter, as this is stiffer (another trick includes putting the catheter in the fridge for a short period of time to make it more stiff).
- *'If that were unsuccessful, I would call a senior for help and advice'.*

Authors' Top Tip

Often students make the mistake of not putting in enough lignocaine jelly. Having done a urology job, it amazes us how this simple piece of advice seems to do the trick most of the time! Be generous with the amount you use, and you will see results.

There are other more stiff urethral catheters available, as well as the suprapubic catheter, but this will usually be performed by a specialist and so is not required for undergraduate finals.

Q3   When would you use a three-way catheter?

(Difficult Question)

- If a patient presented with frank haematuria containing clots. A three-way catheter is used to irrigate the bladder with saline and flush out clots regularly. This is to prevent the patient from going into acute urinary retention, as the clot could potentially block the catheter or the urethra at the bladder neck.
- It is also used post-TURP/TURBT for irrigation purposes, again to prevent the formation of clots that could cause urinary retention.

Q4   It is the middle of the night; you are called by the nurse who says your patient's urine output has dropped suddenly from 70 mL/hour to 10 mL/hour and now zero. What is the most likely cause?

(Difficult Question)

- The most common cause of an apparent drop in urine output in an otherwise well patient is that the catheter is blocked; therefore check it first. This can be done by flushing the catheter and checking to see if you can aspirate the same amount back.

- In some cases (and note that this is not uncommon), the catheter has moved and is not *in situ*. Therefore, when you assess the patient, it is important to look at the bed sheets: you may find the missing urine output soaking into the bed.
- If these options have all been excluded, then you must manage the patient as you would any patient with a drop in urine output. This means taking a focused clinical history, targeting your examination of the abdomen by looking for a distended bladder and reinserting a fresh catheter.
- If the patient truly is oliguric, then you must perform a fluid challenge. (*see* Chapter 8, Initial assessment of a surgical emergency: Case 6.)

Q5 If your catheter pack didn't have a pre-prepared syringe to inflate the balloon, would you use normal saline instead?

(Honours Question)

- Do not use normal saline in the balloon syringe.
- This solution contains crystals that can crystallise and block the syringe port, making it impossible to deflate the balloon, which clearly can be problematic when trying to remove a catheter. Your friendly urologist will not be pleased with you!

Authors' Top Tip

Most catheter packs come with a balloon syringe; if you can't find it, look for it! The normal syringes on the ward will not fit into the balloon port.

Case 2: Simple interrupted suturing of a wound

Instructions: Please suture this wound using a simple interrupted technique.

Introduction
As for any clinical encounter (*see* Chapter 1, Principles of a clinical encounter). Specifically for this case:
✔ **Wash your hands**
✔ **Maintain aseptic technique:** Remember, this procedure needs to be done under sterile conditions, as you have the potential to introduce infection.
✔ **Take a short history:**
- **History of the wound:** Ask the patient how the wound was sustained, particularly if there was any involvement of glass; if this is the case, tell the examiner you would like to X-ray the area for foreign bodies. Glass will show up on plain radiographs, since it is radio-opaque.

- **Assess the need for antibiotics:** If the wound is contaminated, older than 6 hrs or as a result of an animal or a human bite, you need to discuss with a senior before you close the wound. For example, dog bites are generally left to heal by secondary intention or delayed primary intention if they are large, and patients are given broad-spectrum antibiotics. A human bite is a lot more serious, as joint involvement is common and can lead to septic arthritis. Therefore, you should not close this wound; it needs to be dealt with as an emergency by the orthopaedic team. The patient will have to go to theatre for exploration, washout and debridement of the wound; antibiotics are especially important in this case.
- **Tetanus status:** Ask about tetanus booster status; if the patient has not had the booster in the preceding 10 years, then he or she will require one now.

✔ **Prepare your equipment:**

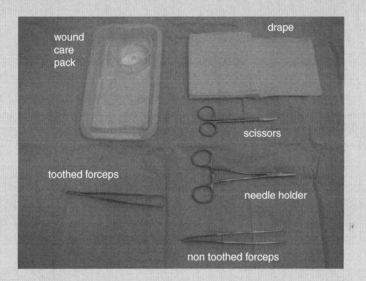

Figure 11.2: Suture pack

- **Open your wound care pack:** This contains a drape, a receptacle for antiseptic solution such as Betadine and gauze.
- **Open your suture pack:** This contains a needle holder, scissors and toothed and non-toothed forceps.
- Select a suitable suture material, e.g. 4/0 non-absorbable and sterile gloves.
- Find two needles, one green to draw up local anaesthetic into a 5-mL syringe and one orange needle to infiltrate with.

The suture material and size you use will depend on the wound site:

Table 11.1: Choice of suture material

Region	Suture material
Limbs	4/0 non-absorbable; remove at 10 days **Hands:** 5/0 non-absorbable; remove at 10 days
Trunk	3/0 non-absorbable; remove at 10 days
Scalp	3/0 non-absorbable; remove at 7 days
Face	5/0 or 6/0 non-absorbable; remove at 3–5 days **Lips/mouth:** 6/0 absorbable

<u>Procedure</u>

✔ **Examine the neurovascular status of the area**
  ■ Examine just distal to the wound for evidence of compromise.
  ■ Normally it is enough to simply say this to the examiner.
✔ **Inspect the wound wearing gloves**
  ■ Examine the wound carefully for any foreign bodies, e.g. glass, debris.
  ■ Irrigate wound with normal saline as needed; often you will need copious amounts.
✔ **Now put on sterile gloves:** Using a no-touch technique
✔ **Drape the area**
  ■ Clean the skin with antiseptic solution, then drape it when dry.
✔ **Apply local anaesthetic**
  ■ Ask your assistant (the examiner) to open a vial of local anaesthetic.
  ■ Draw up to 5 mL in your syringe using the green needle.
  ■ Then, detach the needle without resheathing it and place it straight into the clinical sharps waste bin.

Authors' Top Tip

You must be seen to do this, as there is a mark for disposing of needles safely.

  ■ Attach the orange needle, which will be used to infiltrate the wound.

Authors' Top Tip

Be sure to check the vial before you draw up; review the expiry date and check the solution for its adrenaline content, as adrenaline cannot be used on extremities.

  ■ Infiltrate with the orange needle, aspirating before you inject to prevent you from inadvertently injecting into a blood vessel, which can cause CNS depression, convulsions and cardiac arrhythmias–specifically heart block.

- Give sufficient time for the anaesthetic to work; often this means testing the area with a sharp needle before proceeding.

✔ **Suture the wound**
- Use the simple interrupted method.
- With the toothed forceps, grasp the skin margins and pick them up.
- Apply several sutures 5–10 mm apart; pass the suture needle perpendicular through the skin approximately 1 mm away from the skin edge.
- Pass the needle through the opposite skin edge and tighten to appose the skin edges.
- Now tie the suture into a knot using the instrument tie technique (two complete sutures are enough for the examination); ensure that this is tension free.

Authors' Top Tip

When tying the knot, never handle the suture needle with your fingers; always use the needle holder or forceps to avoid causing an inadvertent needle stick injury and receiving a negative mark on your examination.

✔ **Dress the wound:** E.g. use a non-adhesive dressing.

Completion
✔ **Thank the patient**
✔ **Wash your hands**
✔ **Document the procedure**

'I will give the patient verbal and written wound care advice to go home with and advise the patient to see his or her GP for suture removal in X days time'.

The timing of suture removal depends on the site of the wound and the general health of the patient. Those on steroids may take longer to heal (*see* Table 11.1).

Unfortunately, the only way to get a good grasp of this procedure is to actually practice suturing. The best place is in your hospital clinical skills lab, where you can get a feel for the toughness of the skin pads commonly used in OSCEs. Alternatively, you may find a helpful nurse practitioner in A&E Minors who may give you a demonstration, offer to teach you and observe your technique.

Viva questions

Q1 In what situations would you not use lignocaine with adrenaline?
- When anesthetising extremities, because they are supplied by end arteries. The adrenaline may cause tissue ischaemia and necrosis.

Q2   When would you give a tetanus booster?
- If the patient hasn't had a booster in the last 10 years.
- If the patient is unsure.
- And if the wound is tetanus prone, i.e. contaminated.

Q3   What are the three stages of wound healing?

(Difficult Question)

- Acute inflammatory phase, proliferative phase, maturation phase.

Q4   What is primary and secondary intention in terms of wound healing?

(Difficult Question)

- Primary intention is where the wound edges can be easily approximated and the wound heals by rapid epithelialisation, with minimal granulation and scar tissue.
- Secondary intention is where the wound edges cannot be approximated, so the wound is left open; it then heals from deep within the wound by granulation, epithelialisation and contraction. Healing takes much longer and results in unsightly scars.

Case 3: Nasogastric tube insertion

Instructions: This gentleman has bowel obstruction. Please insert an NG tube.

Introduction
As for any clinical encounter (*see* Chapter 1, Principles of a clinical encounter). Specifically for this case:
✔ **Wash your hands**
✔ **Position the patient appropriately:** Have the patient sit up at the edge of the bed with his neck slightly flexed.
✔ **Prepare your equipment:**
- Open your pack using aseptic technique; ensure you use a wide-bore (16F) NG tube.
- Give the patient a glass of water; this is to aid swallowing as you advance the tube and help with its passage.
- Use aqueous jelly for lubrication; you will also need gauze and local anaesthetic spray.

Procedure
✔ **Approximate your tube length**
- Measure the distance from the patient's nose to the tragus of his ear, then from there to the xiphisternum; mark this distance on the tube.

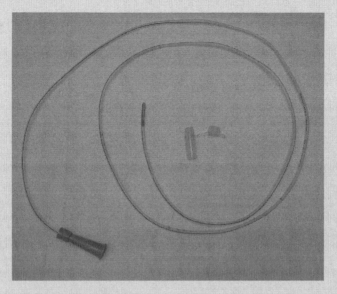

Figure 11.3: Wide-bore NG tube (Ryle's)

- This is the approximate length of tubing you will need to reach the stomach.
✔ **Apply local anaesthetic**
  - Spray the nostril with Xylocaine and wait for its effect for at least five minutes.

Authors' Top Tip

The use of local anaesthetic depends on the tolerance of the patient and the speed of your tube insertion! In the examination, be kind and offer the Xylocaine spray.

✔ **Pass the tube**
  - Ensure the tip is lubricated with aqueous jelly, and gently pass it into the right nostril along its floor into the nasopharynx.
  - Eventually the patient will be able to feel the tube at the back of his throat. At this point, ask him to start taking sips of water and swallow; with each swallow, advance the tube further.
  - Periodically, you can ask the patient to open their mouth and have a look in the oropharynx to make sure you can see the tube and that it is not coiling in the nose or nasopharynx.
✔ **Advance the tube**
  - There is usually very little if any, resistance if the tube is in the oesophagus.
  - If the patient begins to cough, then stop, pull the tube back and reposition.

> ## Authors' Top Tip
>
> *The right nostril is often easier than the left, although if you fail, use the other nostril. We find sometimes it is easier to advance the tube using a rotating movement rather than gently pushing the tube.*

✔ **Confirm correct position**
- **Aspiration test:** Aspirate the stomach contents and confirm acidity with litmus paper.
- **Auscultation:** Inject a small volume of air and listen over the stomach for a rumbling noise; this is called borborygmi.
- **X-ray:** For fine-bore feeding tubes, check the position of the radio-opaque marker on CXR. If the tube is simply being used to drain the contents of the stomach or for decompression purposes in cases of bowel obstruction, an X-ray to check position is not normally required.

Completion
✔ Thank the patient
✔ Wash your hands
✔ Document the procedure

Wide-bore NG tubes are used to aspirate the contents of the stomach. This is commonly used in the treatment of bowel obstruction as part of the 'drip and suck' regimen, routinely in GI surgery or in patients at risk of aspiration, e.g. those post-trauma.

Do not confuse this tube with the fine-bore tube used for enteral feeding purposes. This feeding tube is smaller in calibre (8F) and has a rigid guide wire to aid insertion. As the patient is receiving food or medication enterally, it is crucial that this tube be X-rayed to ensure it is in the correct position. Often, as an FY1 doctor you will be called by the nursing staff for this very reason. Ensure that the radio-opaque marker in the guide wire tip is below the level of the diaphragm, as this suggests it is in the stomach. And if you are unsure, always ask a senior to review the film before the patient starts feeds.

Although this procedure is being increasingly performed by our nursing colleagues, it still remains a popular OSCE station. Remember, if you do insert an NG feeding tube, please do not make the mistake of removing the guide wire before doing the check X-ray!

> ## Authors' Top Tip
>
> *Do not insert an NG tube in cases of suspected basal skull fracture in case the tube inadvertently goes through the fracture into the cranial vault. Also, do not insert an NG tube in patients who have had a recent oesophagectomy, as you do not want to damage a fresh anastomosis.*

Case 4: Chest drain insertion

Instructions: Describe briefly how you would insert a chest drain.

Key features to mention:
- **Consent:** *'I would firstly consent the patient, ensuring that he or she understood the indications and complications of a chest drain and any alternatives to it'.* (*see* Chapter 1, Communication Skills: Case 1.)
- **Check the CXR:** To confirm the pathology (pneumothorax, effusion) and the correct side.
- **Position the patient appropriately:** Ideally, the patient should be seated on a couch at 45° with his or her hands behind the neck on the affected side. This is so that the intercostal spaces become wider.
- **Procedure:**
  - Using aseptic technique, clean and drape the patient. Infiltrate with local anaesthetic into the fifth intercostal space anterior to the mid-axillary line.
  - Make a 2-cm, transverse incision above the rib in the safe triangle (this is to avoid the neurovascular bundle, which lies below the rib).
  - With a haemostat (or blunt dissection scissors), bluntly dissect down to the pleura.
  - Once the pleura is reached, insert a finger into the cavity and sweep away any adhesions; confirm that you are in the thorax.
  - Remove the trocar and insert the chest drain into the cavity using the haemostat as an aid. Guide the tube towards the apex for a pneumothorax or down to the base for an effusion.
  - Tie the drain in place with a suture, ensuring you add a second purse-string suture to be used for skin closure after removal of the drain.
  - Attach the drain to an underwater seal, and ensure the water is bubbling and swinging with each breath. The underwater seal allows air to escape during expiration.
  - Place a sterile dressing over the wound site.
- **Repeat the CXR:** To confirm correct position of the drain.

Completion

Although you would not be expected to perform this procedure for finals, you should be aware of its principles, as you may well be asked to describe the procedure in a viva.

Viva questions

Q1 How would you check if the drain was blocked or not?
- Ask the patient to cough; you should normally see the water bubbling.

Blockage of the tube from kinks or clots will be manifested as a lack of bubbling or a drain that doesn't swing. A persistently bubbling drain suggests a continual leak from the lung.

Q2 What is the safe triangle?

(Difficult Question)

- This is an imaginary area that is deemed 'safe' to insert chest drains.
- The area is bounded by the fourth to the sixth intercostal spaces and the anterior axillary line to the mid-axillary line.
- This is anatomically defined as the anterior border of latissimus dorsi, the lateral border of pectoralis major and a horizontal line through the anatomical position of the ipsilateral nipple.

Q3 Where must you position the underwater seal?

(Difficult Question)

- The underwater seal must be positioned below the level of the patient; this is so the water in the seal doesn't enter the chest.

(Good Response)

- The hydrostatic pressure in the fluid column in the tube will counterbalance the negative pleural pressure and prevent water from being sucked up into the pleural space. If the level of the underwater seal is raised, the fluid column height will be reduced, and as hydrostatic pressure is proportional to this height, water will be sucked into the pleural space.

(Honours Response)

Q4 When would you clamp a chest drain?

(Difficult Question)

- Chest drains that are draining a pleural effusion can be clamped to control the rate of drainage and prevent a life threatening re-expansion pulmonary oedema.
- Chest drains for a pneumothorax should never be clamped; this would create a closed pneumothorax, which would then be at risk of tensioning.

11.2 SURGICAL INSTRUMENTS

This can take the form of a stand-alone OSCE station where you are shown pictures of instruments or surgical equipment and asked to annotate the labels and answer some questions. You will usually be asked for examples of where you have seen the instruments being used. In some medical schools, however, the examiner will hand you an instrument and ask you to tell him or her what it is. In either case, the principles are the same.

Instrument examination

✔ **Name the instrument**
- If you know the correct technical name for the instrument, then say it.
- If you are unsure, use a generic name if possible, e.g. if you are handed a Debakey vascular clamp, just say: *'This is a surgical clamp'.*
- If you are really stuck, describe the instrument as much as you can.

Examiner's Anecdote

'He described the instrument almost flawlessly, even though he didn't know its surgical name. It was like watching the "Antiques Roadshow", and he was selling me the instrument! Even if you don't know the eponymous names, describe what you see and you will score well'.

Authors' Top Tip

In some cases, students may not know the name of the instrument but have seen it being used during a procedure; here, it is acceptable to tell the examiner that you do not know the actual name; instead, discuss where you have seen it being used, that way you can still score some points.

Most of the instruments will be common things you will see in clinical practice. But prepare yourself for anything; one of the authors was handed a laparoscopic port in finals.

✔ **Indications for use**
- Give examples of where you have seen the instruments being used, preferably during surgery in an area of which you are familiar. (This can only work in your favour, as the examiner is then likely to ask you about the example you give.)

  e.g. *'This is a laparoscopic port. I have seen it used in a laparoscopic cholecystectomy in a patient who had suffered multiple bouts of biliary colic and acute cholecystitis …'*

This way you have placed the onus on the examiner to ask you about gallstone disease, or if laparoscopic surgery is your forte, you can even discuss this.

As there are many possible examples from which to choose, in the cases described below, we offer examples of discussions that you may wish to use to prepare for your examinations.

✔ **Describe the associated procedure**
- Tell the examiner how to use the instrument in clinical practice.

  e.g. *'This is a chest drain. I have seen this used in the management of a polytrauma patient suffering from a pneumothorax. The chest drain is inserted into the safe triangle on the affected side by first making a 2-cm, transverse incision above the rib and bluntly dissecting down to the pleura …' (see* Surgical procedures, Case 4)

In the above example, the examiner may ask you the indications for chest drain insertion, its complications, management or even the anatomical boundaries of the safe triangle. The examiner may even ask you the emergency management of a tension pneumothorax or to discuss ATLS principles; the possibilities are endless! We have seen top students who have begun such a viva and gone on to discuss the British Thoracic Society (BTS) guidelines on chest drain management and removal. Work towards your strengths; the examiner will only be impressed with your knowledge.

Completion

Students often say the instrument station is meaningless, and they don't see how it can even last the length of a standard five-minute OSCE station.

However, some students may be offered more than one instrument in this station. Often the reason for this is that the candidate's initial response was poor or minimal, and the examiner is simply trying to help the candidate score as many points as possible. But from the above examples you can see how a simple instrument can lead to a viva discussion between you and the examiner, where you are demonstrating your breath and depth of knowledge. Take this as an opportunity for you to shine.

Case 1: Intravenous cannulae

Instructions: What is this instrument, and can you tell me where you have seen this being used?

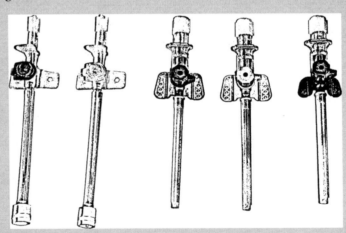

Figure: 11.4 Cannulae

- This is a multiple array of intravenous cannulae, ranging in size from small to large bore. The colour is an indicator of the tube radius; blue is the smallest and brown or grey is the largest.
- **Indications:** A cannula is used in any surgical emergency for resuscitation purposes, immediate decompression of tension pneumothorax and normal daily fluid replacement.

- **Procedure:** Discuss how to insert a peripheral venous cannula.
- **Viva discussion:** Discuss emergency management of any surgical patient (*see* Chapter 8).

Viva questions

Q1   Do any laws govern the flow rate in a blood vessel?

(Honours Question)

- The flow rate of a liquid through a tubular structure is proportional to the fourth power of the radius and inversely proportional to the length and viscosity (Poiseuille's law).
- Hence, large-bore cannulae are short in length and have far greater flow rates.
- According to the principle, a small increase in the radius will lead to a large increase in flow rate. This means if you double the radius, the flow rate will increase to the power of four, i.e. 16 times.
- This is why large-bore cannulae are preferred in the emergency setting, as they are able to deliver a large volume of fluid quickly.

Authors' Top Tip

Do not underestimate the importance of this procedure; the insertion of an intravenous cannula has even been examined in the most recent postgraduate MRCS examination.

Case 2: Intravenous fluids

Instructions: What are these, and where have you seen them being used?

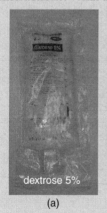 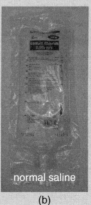 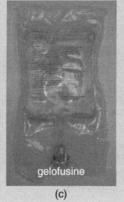 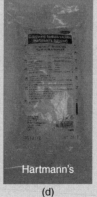

| dextrose 5% | normal saline | gelofusine | Hartmann's |
| (a) | (b) | (c) | (d) |

Figure 11.5a, b, c, d: Intravenous fluids

- This is a multiple array of intravenous fluids, crystalloids (normal saline, Hartmann's and dextrose) and colloids (Gelofusine).
- **Indications:** They are used to replace normal daily fluid requirements, for resuscitation purposes and for fluid challeges.
- **Viva discussion:** Discuss the assessment of fluid status, resuscitation and fluid challenge in post-operative oliguria or hypotension in a polytrauma patient (*see* Chapter 8).

Viva questions

Q1   How does the fluid in the above intravenous fluids redistribute in the body?

(Difficult Question)

Table 11.2: Fluid distribution

Fluid	Example	Distribution
Water (hypotonic)	Dextrose (5%)	This distributes throughout the whole body water. Only 7.5% will remain in the intravascular compartment.
Crystalloid (isotonic)	Normal saline, Hartmann's, Ringer's lactate	Fluid distributes in the ECF. Twenty-one per cent will remain in the intravascular compartment.
Colloid	Gelofusine, albumin	Fluid distributes in the intravascular compartment and almost all of it stays there, as the membrane is impermeable.

- In clinical practice, the distribution properties of these fluids requires that large volumes of water, less volume of crystalloids and an even smaller volume of colloid is needed to result in the same corresponding rise in plasma volume.

The total body water content is approximately 45 L in a 70-kg male, one third of which is extracellular fluid (ECF); the remaining two thirds is intracellular fluid (ICF). The plasma constitutes 21% of the ECF space; plasma overall constitutes approximately 7.5% of total body water.

Q2   What is the fundamental difference between crystalloids and colloids?

(Difficult Question)

A *crystalloid* is an electrolyte solution in water; this forms a true solution that can diffuse through a semi-permeable membrane.

   A *colloid* is a fluid that contains high-molecular-weight molecules that do not pass through a semi-permeable membrane. This does not form a true solution.

(Surgical Definition)

■ As colloids cannot diffuse through a semi-permeable membrane, they remain in the intravascular compartment longer. They can be natural or synthetic in origin, and so there is an associated theoretical risk of anaphylaxis.
■ There is much controversy with regards to what is the ideal fluid for resuscitation purposes. There are points for and against either fluid type; in the United Kingdom, however, crystalloids are generally used in the acute setting for resuscitation.

Q3 What is third-space loss?

(Difficult Question)

■ Fluid is distributed into three spaces: the ICF space, the ECF space and a 'third' space.
■ This third space is pathological and is usually fluid sequestration due to some underlying disease process; it often leads to significant dehydration and is commonly seen in pancreatitis and bowel obstruction.
■ This is an important feature to remember when monitoring fluid balance on input and output charts, as you will need to estimate this 'third-space loss' through other means, i.e. clinical examination.

Q4 What is the normal daily fluid requirement?

Table 11.3: Normal fluid balance

Input (mL)	Output (mL)
Oral fluids: 1 500	**Sensible losses**
Food: 1 000	**Urine:** 1 500
Metabolic: 350	**Faeces:** 300
	Insensible losses
	Lungs: 500
	Skin: 550
Total: 2 850 mL	**Total: 2 850 mL**

■ Therefore, an average male adult who leads a sedentary lifestyle will require approximately 3 L of fluid per day as a normal requirement.
■ Various fluid replacement regimes aim to achieve this balance, e.g. 2 L of 5% dextrose and 1 L normal saline often with supplemental potassium in the form of potassium chloride (KCL). In a 70-kg man, this equates up to 70 mmol in three divided doses daily.
■ **Daily Na requirement:** 1–1.5 mmol/kg; **Daily K requirement:** 1 mmol/kg
■ After non-cardiac surgery, K^+ supplementation is avoided in the first 24 hours. K^+ levels rise post surgery as a result of damage to tissues and cells, the release of K^+ during surgery and the consequent 'stress' response due to the trauma from the operation.

Case 3: Suture material

Instructions: What is this, and can you tell me where you have seen it being used?

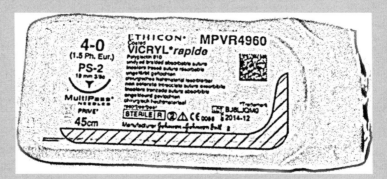

Figure 11.6: Vicryl

- This is 4/0 Vicryl, which is a synthetic, absorbable, braided suture material.
- **Indications:** The material is used in bowel anastomosis and tying pedicles.
- **Viva discussion:** Discuss how to suture a wound (*see* Surgical procedures, Case 2).

Viva Questions

Q1 How do you classify suture materials?

(Difficult Question)

- In general, sutures can be either synthetic or natural (e.g. silk) and can be further classified into monofilament or braided.

Table 11.4: Suture material

Suture class	Description
Absorbable	**Natural:** Catgut (theoretical risk of prion disease; rarely used) **Synthetic monofilament:** Monocryl (subcuticular skin closure); Polydioxanone (PDS) (abdominal wall closure) **Synthetic braided:** Dexon; Vicryl
Non-absorbable	**Natural:** Silk (securing drains) **Synthetic monofilament:** Prolene (vascular anastomoses); Ethilon (skin wound closure); steel (sternotomy closure) **Synthetic braided:** Silk

The size of the suture is based on the '0' system, where the finer the diameter of the suture, the greater the number preceding the '0', e.g. 6/0 is thinner than 3/0. Monofilament sutures are slippery, whereas braided sutures can provide more secure knots but have a theoretical risk of infection forming between the strands. Synthetic sutures tend to return to their original straight state; that is they have 'memory', which makes knot tying technically more difficult. Silk has almost no memory so is an ideal suture for knot tying.

Case 4: Forceps

Instructions: What are these, and can you tell me where you have seen them being used?

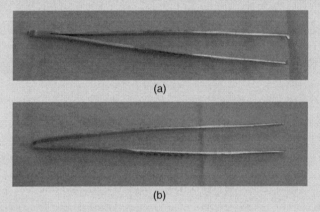

(a)

(b)

Figure 11.7: (a) Toothed forceps; (b) Non-toothed forceps

- These are toothed and non-toothed forceps used for grasping and handling tissues.

Table 11.5: Forceps

Forceps	Description
Toothed forceps	▪ These have at least one tooth on one tip that interdigitates with two teeth on the opposing tip.
	▪ They provide good traction as the teeth puncture the tissues and also provide grip by tethering, thereby preventing slippage.
	▪ Toothed forceps are useful in cases where you need to handle tough tissue like skin, which tolerates puncture but not compression.
	▪ The tethering effect of the forceps is useful when handling slippery tissues such as fascia and bone.
Non-toothed Forceps	▪ These atraumatic forceps have serrations on the opposing tips in order to maintain grip.
	▪ They are used for handling delicate tissues, e.g. bowel or blood vessels. Toothed forceps should not be used in these situations, as puncture will lead to content leakage.
	▪ They are also useful for holding and tying sutures.

Case 5: Antiseptic solution

Instructions: What are these? Can you tell me where you have seen them being used?

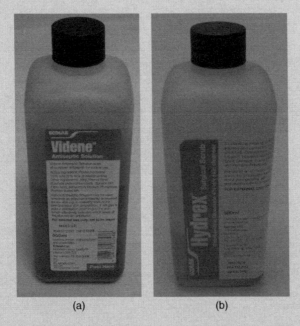

(a)   (b)

Figure 11.8: (a) Betadine; (b) Chlorhexidine

- These are two antiseptic solutions: Betadine and chlorhexidine.
- **Indications:** They are used as antiseptic for skin preparation and surgical hand scrubbing preoperatively.
- **Viva discussion:** 'Scrubbing up' *(see below)*.

Viva questions

Q1 How do you wash your hands ('scrub up') in preparation for surgery?
- 'Scrubbing up' involves: hand washing, gowning and gloving; it takes 2–3 minutes.

Prepare your equipment
- Select a surgical gown pack; unwrap the pack and place its contents onto the drape provided on top of a trolley.
- Select a suitably sized sterile glove; unwrap the pack and place its contents onto the sterile field created by the drape.

- Ensure you have your clogs, theatre scrubs, theatre cap, face mask and/or eye protection (goggles) on already.
- Remove all jewellery, including watches.

Hand washing

- Keep your hands above elbow level at all times.
- **Turn on the tap:** Adjust to a comfortable temperature and rate to avoid splashing.
- **Wash your hands:** Dispense antiseptic solution onto your palms using the elbow lever.
  - Rub your hands palm to palm.
  - Then, rub the dorsum of your left hand with the palm of your right.
  - Now, rub hands palm to palm with your fingers interlaced.
  - Rub the back of your fingers with the palm of the opposing hand; keep your fingers interlocked.
  - Rub the thumb by grasping it with the thumb and index finger of your opposing hand and gently rotating.
  - Clasp the fingers of the opposing hand and rub the palms.

Remember to repeat all manoeuvres on the opposite hand.

- **Wash the forearm:** Both forearms are lathered up to the elbows using the opposite hand and moving up circumferentially from the wrist; in the last cycle, wash up to one third from the elbow.
- **Rinse off the suds and repeat up to three times:** Remember to keep your hands above elbow level so that the dirty effluent runs down off the elbows and not back over your hands.
- **Turn off the taps:** Using your elbows.
- **Dry your hands:** Use the two towels provided in the gown pack; one for each arm. Pat the skin dry, working up towards the elbows.

Gowning

- Once your hands are dry, pinch the gown from the inside at the shoulder tips and lift it off the sterile field, holding it away from your body.
- The gown should be allowed to drop open in front of you; ensure that the gown is high enough that it doesn't touch the floor.
- As the gown is unfolded, place your arms through the sleeves and make sure your hands do not exit the holes beyond the cuff (if they do, they will touch the outside of the gown, and this will desterilise it).
- An assistant will tie your gown from behind; to complete the waist strap, you must have already put on your sterile gloves, so your assistant will help you tie this.

Gloving

- Use a 'no touch' technique; this means your hands should not touch the outside surface of the gloves at any point when putting them on.

Always keep your hands above waist level and if they are not in use, keep them folded.

11.3 MISCELLANEOUS PROCEDURES AND INSTRUMENTS FOR FINALS

Table 11.6: Other procedures

Procedure	Description
Intramuscular injection (IM)	**Indication:** This is used to deliver medications, e.g. analgesia or sedation. **Equipment:** 21G *(green needle)* or 23G *(blue needle)*. **Area of injection:** The deltoid, lateral thigh or upper outer quadrant of the buttock (to avoid the sciatic nerve). **Procedure:** Draw up the medication with the green needle and attach the injecting needle, e.g. the 21G, for buttock injection. Wipe the area with an alcohol swab. Insert the needle perpendicular to the skin and draw back, ensuring you are not in a blood vessel, and slowly inject the medication. Withdraw the needle and wipe the puncture site with cotton wool.
Subcutaneous injection (SC)	**Indication:** This is used to deliver medications, e.g. insulin, heparin. **Equipment:** 25G *(orange needle)*. **Area of injection:** Skin folds, e.g. the forearm or abdomen. **Procedure:** Draw up the medication with the green needle and attach the 25G injecting needle. Wipe the area with an alcohol swab. Pinch the skin and gently lift into a fold; insert the needle horizontally into the skin fold, drawing back as necessary to ensure you are not in a vein. Inject slowly and withdraw when complete, then wipe puncture site with cotton wool.

Table 11.7: Other instruments

Equipment	Description
Drains	**Indications:** Drains are used to divert fluid from a blockage, decompress, minimise dead space in a wound to prevent fluid from collecting, to drain actual fluid collections or monitor/protect an anastomosis at risk of leaking. **Equipment:** Drains can be either open or closed systems. A closed system is one that has a container. They can be further divided into active or passive systems. An active system applies suction, allowing better drainage but risking damage to surrounding structures; whereas a passive system allows drainage by gravity. **Passive open, e.g.** Penrose or corrugated drains. **Passive closed, e.g.** chest drain, urinary catheter, Robinson. **Active closed, e.g.** Redivac (vacuum drain).
Sterile pack	**Indications:** These packs are used in any general procedure requiring sterility, e.g. when cleaning a wound, suturing. **Equipment:** The pack contains a dressing towel, a two-compartment tray with non-woven swaps, a 60 mL gallipot receptacle for solution and disposable forceps, sterile gloves, a yellow clinical waste bag, a sterile laminate sheet to act as a drape and a larger laminate sheet to create a sterile field.

CHAPTER 12

Surgical radiology

Undoubtedly you will spend a great proportion of your house officer years in the radiology department, where your negotiation skills and ability to compromise are tested to their very limits. Radiologists are often given the unfair label of being unreasonable, always saying 'no' to that feeble request for a 'semi-urgent, maybe could wait until tomorrow, but only if you think so, CT scan!' But surgeons often work very closely with radiologists; you may notice consultant radiologists at your weekly MDT meetings, advising on the operative plan of action. As a junior doctor, you will often discuss scan results with radiologists, usually at times when they themselves are busy reporting other scans. Having a basic knowledge of the various image modalities available and the key features you are looking for will not only give you good grounds to make your case for your patient, but will also place you highly in the mind of your friendly radiologist!

Our goal is not to teach you to review images like a radiologist; that is beyond the scope of this book and is certainly not required for finals. However, you must bear in mind that a surgeon encounters a wide variety of image modalities in his or her day-to-day clinical practice, and accurate interpretation of those images will in some cases determine the treatment plans for the patients under your care. As a house officer, you will be the one asked to request these images and will probably be the first team member to review them.

Authors' Top Tip

Depending on your hospital, plain-film radiographs may not be immediately reported, and so it is important you have a good understanding of how to interpret them as well as be able to spot any gross pathology.

The most common image modality you will come across in the hospital setting is the plain-film radiograph. It is highly likely, therefore, that you will be presented with a chest or abdominal radiograph during your final clinical examinations. Here, we will discuss a common approach when addressing the plain radiograph presented to you during your examination to help you to achieve the maximum available marks. It has been noted that some medical schools have a separate OSCE station devoted entirely for this purpose. Increasingly, more technical image modalities are being assessed during finals, not so much to test your understanding of the radiological principles, but to assess your ability to detect obvious gross pathology, which in the examination can act as a starting point for further clinically orientated viva discussions.

In most cases, you are simply given an image and asked to comment on it with minimal – if any – history at all. We feel this makes the case unrealistic, as in clinical practise you would often have some form of history, even if it's just a brief handover from the ambulance crew. If you find yourself stuck, it is perfectly acceptable to ask for any further history that you feel may assist you in your diagnosis. However, in the examination it is likely that any additional history will not be available, and so the examiner will ask you to proceed. But do not be flustered by this; the diagnosis may only be one mark, so remain cool and carry on with your systematic examination. The examiners are looking for confident and competent individuals.

Authors' Top Tip

Avoid the use of the word 'X-ray', as technically you cannot see X-rays but can see the resultant radiographic image. We advise using the word 'radiograph' instead.

General principles of image reporting

To begin describing any piece of imaging, always start with the basics.

✔ **Image details**
  - **Patient details:** Identify the patient's name, gender and age.
  - **Image details:** This includes the date the image was taken. You can also state whether it is a supine or erect film (this will normally be marked on the radiograph).

✔ **Assess the technical quality of the radiograph**
  - **Projection:** Identify whether it is an AP (i.e. film behind the patient, X-ray machine in front of the patient), PA (i.e. film in front of the patient), lateral or oblique film.
  - **Orientation:** Identify the left and right sides of the film; there will normally be a marker on the film with an 'R' on the right and an 'L' on the left side of the film.
  - **Rotation:** This depends on the film, e.g. in a CXR the medial ends of the clavicles should be equidistant from the spinous vertebral processes that fall between them.
  - **Penetration:** If bone is too clearly visible, then the film is overpenetrated; if you cannot see the bony structures clearly, then it is underpenetrated.
  - **Degree of inspiration (for CXR interpretation):** There should be six anterior ribs or 10 posterior ribs visible to the level of the diaphragm. If a greater number are visible, then the lung fields are hyper-inflated, if fewer are visible, then there has been a less-than-normal inspiratory effort. A poor inspiratory effort can give the misleading appearance of cardiomegaly and basal shadowing when there is no actual pathology. This is commonly seen in patients who are unable to take a deep breath either due to pain or lung pathology such as pneumonia.

The basic densities that will be visible on a plain radiograph include:

Table 12.1: Image densities

Structure	Image density
Gas	Black
Fat	Dark grey
Soft tissue/fluid	Light grey
Bone/calcification	White
Metal	Intense white

Specific image evaluation

- Follow your systematic routine for evaluating each image modality.

Some candidates go for the most obvious pathology first; although this is acceptable, you must remember to go back and evaluate the whole radiograph systematically, as you do not want to miss out on more subtle abnormalities. For purposes of clarity, the cases in this chapter will be described using the former approach.

Completion

Once you have summarised your findings to the examiner, offer a differential diagnosis. We suggest you use this opportunity to start a viva discussion. In some cases, the topic for discussion will be obvious, e.g. if you diagnose bowel obstruction, the examiner will most likely ask you how to manage it. In some medical schools, however, there are standardised set of questions that in many cases are fairly predictable.

Authors' Top Tip

Preempt the examiner and start the viva discussion yourself; this not only demonstrates your confidence but gives you the added advantage of directing the viva, allowing you to concentrate on your strong areas.

Reporting the plain-film chest radiograph

✔ **General principles** (*as above*)
✔ **Examine the lung fields**
- Compare the size; they will be reduced in collapse.
- Look for discrete opacities; compare one side to the other.
- Compare transradiancy. They should be the same colour; if one is whiter than the other, this suggests fluid as seen in a haemothorax or effusion. If one is blacker, this may indicate a pneumothorax.
✔ **Check the hilum**
- Compare shape and density; remember the left will be higher than the right.

✔ **Assess the heart**
  ▪ The normal width should be less than half of the transthoracic diameter. However, in an AP film you cannot comment on this, as the heart is falsely enlarged. Comment on shape as well as size.
  ▪ Identify the heart borders. Any blurring may suggest consolidation.
✔ **Look at the diaphragm**
  ▪ Normally, right is higher than the left, as it is pushed up by the liver. A very high position may suggest a diaphragmatic hernia.
  ▪ Look at the area under the diaphragm for a rim of air that is seen in the perforation of a hollow viscus within the abdominal cavity.
✔ **Examine the costophrenic angles**
  ▪ These should be sharp and clear.
  ▪ They may be blunted in the presence of an effusion, haemothorax, consolidation or collapse.
✔ **Identify the mediastinum**
  ▪ This should be centrally placed; it may be shifted in an effusion or pneumothorax.
✔ **Assess for tracheal deviation**
✔ **Look at the bones**
  ▪ Examine the vertebrae, ribs and scapulae for any decreased density or signs of fractures.
✔ **Look at soft tissues**
  ▪ There may be pockets of air (surgical emphysema) or swelling.

Reporting the abdominal radiograph

In some adults, one film is not enough to visualise the entire abdomen from the diaphragm to the groin. As a result, you may be presented with two films.

Authors' Top Tip

In a woman of child-bearing age, you must first exclude pregnancy before requesting an abdominal X-ray.

✔ **General principles** *(as above)*
✔ **Check the viscera**
  ▪ Inspect the outline of the organs, making sure they are on the correct side of the film, e.g. liver on the right, spleen on the left. Any structure outlined by gas will be part of the gastrointestinal tract.
  ▪ Also comment on whether the organs appear too big, too small, distorted, contain calculi or gas, e.g. air in the biliary tree.
  ▪ **Small bowel:** This will be in the middle of the radiograph; when it is distended, the valvulae conniventes crossing the entire lumen will be visible. Normally, it should not be greater than 2.5–3 cm in diameter.

- **Large bowel:** This can be differentiated from the small bowel by haustra; these only partly cross the bowel lumen. Normally, large bowel is present around the edges at the periphery of the film.

✔ **Check for normal gas patterns**
  - Look for the normal gastric air bubble.
  - Look for air in the rectum and the presence of faecal matter in the colon.

✔ **Check for any calcification**
  - Pelvic phleboliths, appendicolith.
  - Abdominal aorta or of the iliac arteries (this may be mistaken for an aneurysm if tortuous); you can occasionally see calcification of the splenic artery.
  - Renal, bladder or ureteric calculi.
  - Costal cartilages, calcified lymph nodes (these might change in position from film to film).

✔ **Assess the bony structures**
  - Examine the spine, pelvis and sacroiliac joints.
  - Look for any degenerative changes, cortical thickening, osteoporosis, sclerosis or malignant change (metastases, Paget's disease, myeloma).

There will be differences when the abdominal X-ray is taken in the erect position, as air will rise and fluid will sink. Most of the organs will drop, except the liver and spleen, which are fixed.

The erect film will show fluid levels, an important finding in bowel obstruction. In addition, the X-ray may show a pneumoperitoneum with air under the diaphragm, i.e. evidence of a visceral perforation.

Case 1: Pneumothorax

Instructions: This man was brought into the resus department after having been stabbed in the chest. Comment on his X-ray.

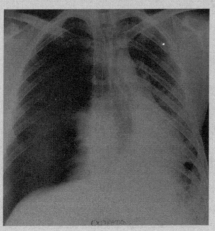

Figure 12.1: Pneumothorax

Key features to note:

- *'This is an AP chest radiograph of Patient X, taken on Date X.*
- *The most obvious abnormality is that of a left-sided pneumothorax, leading to tracheal and mediastinal shift to the opposite side.*
- *This is a **surgical emergency** and requires immediate decompression with a large-bore cannula inserted into the second intercostal space, mid-clavicular line, on the affected side'.*

Completion

- *'In summary, this is a chest radiograph demonstrating a tension pneumothorax. I believe this X-ray should **not** have been taken, as this is a clinical diagnosis and ideally should be detected during the Breathing stage of ATLS principles'.*

(Honours Response)

- *'After immediate decompression with thoracocentesis, the patient requires a chest drain'.*

By ending your presentation at this point, you are left open to discuss a number of different issues that the examiner may ask you as part of the viva. To prevent being caught out, you can take the initiative and continue discussing the emergency management of the patient. The more ambitious candidate may choose to briefly discuss the insertion of a chest drain (*see* Chapter 11, Surgical procedures).

   If the case demonstrates obvious pathology that requires emergency treatment, be sure to emphasise this in your answer. Discussing heart size in the above chest film of a patient with a tension pneumothorax will not stand well with the examiner, who is looking to see how you would deal with this patient when and if you saw such a film. Any consultant who walked into the resus department and saw you examining the above film would first ask you if you had already treated the patient. The examiners are not there to assess your detailed X-ray interpretation skills; they are far more interested in your knowledge of emergencies and their management. It is also important to remember that the examiner would like to sense urgency in your answer; however, demonstrate this in a calm and controlled manner.

Authors' Top Tip

We suggest you spell out the urgency of the situation by using the phrase, 'This is a surgical emergency' first, and then discussing your management thereafter in a step-by-step and logical manner, i.e. what you would actually do in clinical practice.

Ensure you follow ATLS or ALS protocols, as appropriate. After the immediate emergency has been managed, you can go back and take a closer look at the film for other pathology.

Case 2: Oesophageal carcinoma   (Difficult Case)

Instructions: This elderly man presented with dysphagia. Comment on this film.

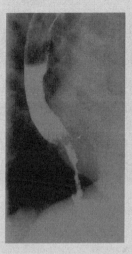

Figure 12.2: Barium swallow

Key features to note:
- *'This is a barium swallow of Patient X, taken on Date X.*
- *The most obvious abnormality is that of a stricture at the distal third of the oesophagus, leading to a shouldered appearance.*
- *This is most likely to be an oesophageal carcinoma'.*

Completion

Oesophageal cancers occur most commonly in the distal third. This is due to an increased incidence of adenocarcinoma as a result of Barrett's oesophagus.

Barium swallow is the best initial test of choice, but OGD is the diagnostic test of choice. It characteristically shows a stricture (similar to the apple-core lesion in the bowel) and is sometimes called a 'shouldered' appearance. The most common differential diagnosis is achalasia, which can look very similar with its so-called 'bird's beak appearance'. To differentiate, the size of the proximally dilated oesophagus is taken into account; with oesophageal cancer progression is so rapid that the dilatation is less than with achalasia. Achalasia tends to affect the distal third, whereas oesophageal cancer can affect any third. In achalasia, there is absence of the gastric air bubble on CXR.

Other possible images you may be shown in the examination are oesophageal varices. Typically, the patient presents with an upper GI bleed and his or her barium swallow demonstrates multiple 'worm-like' filling defects throughout the entire course of the oesophagus. You should be prepared to discuss the management of upper GI bleeding as a surgical emergency.

Case 3: Extradural haematoma

Instructions: This man was involved in an RTA. Comment on his scan.

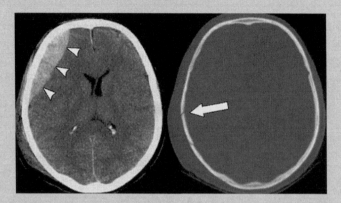

Figure 12.3: CT head

Key features to note:

- *'This is a non-contrast CT head of Patient X, taken on Date X. There is only a single slice.*
- *The most obvious abnormality is a biconvex (or lens-shaped) area of high attenuation over the right frontal region; this is most likely to be blood'.*

(Average Response)

- *'There is no obvious midline shift.*
- *I would like to look at the bone windows setting to check for an associated skull fracture.* [The examiner shows you the image on the right.]
- *Looking at the bone windows, I can see there is a fracture in the parietal bone'.*

(Honours Response)

Completion

- *'In summary, this patient has an extradural haematoma on the right, most likely as a result of trauma.*
- *This is a surgical emergency, and I would manage the patient according to ATLS guidelines'.*

Viva questions

Q1 What is the most common site of bleeding in an extradural haematoma?
- The middle meningeal artery is often lacerated, as it is adjacent to the thin pterion bone; this bone is vulnerable to skull fractures.

Q2   How would you distinguish between an extradural and subdural hematoma?

Table 12.2: Intracranial haematoma

Examination	Extradural	Subdural
History	Classically, there is a period of lucency followed by a fall in GCS.	Patients present with trauma. The elderly are particularly susceptible to this.
CT scan	High attenuation biconvex area; does not cross suture lines.	A crescentic area of high attenuation; can cross suture lines.

Q3   How do you assess the Glasgow Coma Scale (GCS)?

Table 12.3: The Glasgow Coma Scale

Component	GCS score
Eyes	**4** Opens eyes spontaneously. **3** Opens eyes to voice. **2** Opens eyes to pain. **1** No response.
Verbal	**5** Orientated. **4** Talking but confused. **3** Inappropriate speech. **2** Incomprehensible speech. **1** No response.
Movement	**6** Obeys command. **5** Localises to pain. **4** Withdraws from pain. **3** Flexor response (decorticate posture). **2** Extensor response (decerebrate). **1** No response.

The minimum GCS score is 3, and the maximum is 15. Patients with a GCS score of <8 are unable to maintain their airway and therefore require an airway adjunct, usually in the form of a cuffed endotracheal tube.

Authors' Top Tip

Patients with an extradural haematoma may initially have a normal examination. It is therefore important to repeat your neurological examination in all patients with head injuries. The importance of accurately documenting the GCS cannot be underestimated!

Q4   How would you manage this patient?

As the patient is likely to have sustained his injury through trauma, this patient should be managed according to ATLS principles. Although the main concern is a head injury, a poorly controlled airway is more likely to kill a patient far quicker than the haematoma and should be managed first. Do not therefore jump to state you would treat the patient with a Burr hole without having discussed your initial assessment! In reality, there is a trauma team whose purpose is to expedite the primary survey, and as a result many things are done simultaneously.

'As part of my primary survey, I will resuscitate the patient by:
- Ensuring the Airway is patent with adequate Cervical **spine** immobilisation.
- Assessing the patient's Breathing and addressing the patient's Circulation by inserting two large-bore cannulae, one into each antecubital fossa, whilst taking blood for further investigation and a G&S at the same time.
- At this point I would call for senior help and advice, but generally this will include urgently referring the patient to the neurosurgical team for consideration of operative management (a burr hole or craniotomy)'.

This patient has suffered a primary brain injury, i.e. injury sustained at the time of the incident. The aim of the trauma team should be to minimise any secondary brain injury caused by hypoxia, hypercapnia and hypotension.

At this stage in your career, you would not be expected to know the finer details of severe head injury management. However, being aware of the principles can only work in your favour! In general, the patient should be intubated and ventilated (GCS <8); maintained at normocapnia, prescribed prophylactic antibiotics in the case of open-skull fractures and given intravenous mannitol after consultation with neurosurgery, who may decide to take the patient to theatre for urgent evacuation of the haematoma.

This generally completes the primary survey, but in some cases the secondary survey, a thorough top-to-tail examination, may not be completed until a few days later, once the patient has been stabilised and extubated. The purpose of this is to identify any non-life-threatening injuries that could be managed once the immediate threat to life has been treated.

If you are not in a specialist neurosurgical centre, the patient should be immediately transferred to the nearest centre without delay. Imaging the head should not delay transfer; imaging can be performed at the receiving hospital if intracranial pathology is suspected.

Authors' Top Tip

Although we have previously advised you not to 'refer' patients in a viva discussion as, technically speaking, you are the surgical team, ATLS principles insist on urgent transfer or referral to a dedicated neurosurgical centre in cases of suspected head injury. You must get this point across in your viva.

Case 4: Pneumoperitoneum

Instructions: This man presented with abdominal pain. Comment on his film.

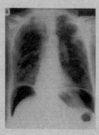

Figure 12.4: Air under the diaphragm

Key features to note:

- *'This is an erect chest radiograph of Patient X, taken on Date X.*
- *The most obvious abnormality is that of air under both hemi diaphragms.*
- *This is most likely due to a perforated intra-abdominal viscus ...'*

(Average Response)

- *The above, plus: 'of which the most common cause is a perforated duodenal ulcer on the anterior part of D1, the first part of the duodenum'.*

(Honours Response)

Authors' Top Tip

This is a classical case for which you should not wait for the examiner to ask you what you will do next. He is likely to ask you for your management! Therefore, preempt the examiner by continuing to talk and discuss your management. He or she may interrupt to ask you further questions or change the direction of the viva. But in most cases, the examiner will be happy to sit back and listen. This shows you are dictating the examination situation and thereby doing better than an average student!

Completion

- *'This is a surgical emergency; I would like to resuscitate the patient, ensure that his airway is patent and secure, check that his breathing is adequate and assess his circulation by inserting two large-bore cannulae, one into each antecubital fossa, whilst taking blood for further investigation at the same time.*
- *I will then begin the patient on aggressive fluid resuscitation, as he is likely to have suffered significant third-space loss.*
- *At this point, I will call for senior help and advice'.*

We suggest you continue your discussion by offering the following answers. For purposes of clarity we provide these as viva questions.

Viva questions

Q1 What investigations would you request?
- FBC, U&Es, clotting, amylase, ABG.
- CX the patient for at least four units of blood in case he requires an operation.

Q2 What would be your further management?
- *'After initiating aggressive fluid resuscitation, I will proceed by inserting a nasogastric tube, a urinary catheter and ideally a central venous line.*
- *The patient will need to be kept NBM and given sufficient pain relief in accordance with the WHO analgesic ladder.*

■ *I will then begin the patient on empirical intravenous antibiotics in accordance with local hospital guidelines or after discussion with a microbiologist'.*

Authors' Top Tip

If the examiner probes and asks which antibiotics you would prescribe, always respond by saying you will follow local hospital antibiotic guidelines, followed by expert advice from a microbiologist. Failing that, you can start a broad-spectrum antibiotic empirically based on your clinical diagnosis.

The empirical antibiotics that have been used traditionally for bowel sepsis are Cefuroxime and Metronidazole, but due to fears of C. difficile (causing pseudo-membranous colitis), this is falling out of favour. Also, there is little evidence to support the use of Metronidazole.

The specific management of a patient with a perforated peptic ulcer can be divided into conservative or surgical measures:

Conservative

■ Some patients respond to conservative treatment when the omentum heals spontaneously; however, most patients go onto surgical management.

Surgical

■ Management of a patient with a perforated peptic ulcer typically involves one of three methods, specifically a laparotomy and wash out with:
   1 An omental patch repair (Graham's method).
   2 Excision of the ulcer.
   3 Gastrectomy (which can be total or partial).

Q3 Do you know of any other causes of air under the diaphragm?

(Honours Question)

■ There are many causes of air under the diaphragm, including, perforation of any intra-abdominal viscus.
   – The most common cause is a perforated ulcer on the anterior part of D1.
   – In addition, the large bowel can perforate secondary to colorectal carcinoma or diverticular disease.
   – Perforation of any intra-abdominal viscus can occur secondary to blunt or penetrating abdominal trauma.
■ This could also be a normal post-operative finding in any patient who has undergone abdominal surgery, most commonly post-laparotomy or laparoscopy, due to air entering the abdominal cavity.

It also occurs in patients post-peritoneal dialysis; in any patient with an intra-abdominal infection with gas-forming bacteria; through air bubbles in a female post-coital (rare); and during waterskiing.

Case 5: Endoscopic retrograde cholangiopancreatogram (ERCP)

Instructions: This gentleman presented with colicky abdominal pain. Comment on his film.

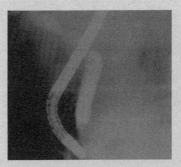

Figure 12.5: ERCP

Key features to note:
- *'This is an endoscopic retrograde cholangiopancreatogram (ERCP) of Patient X, taken on Date X.*
- *The most obvious abnormality is that of a filling defect at the distal end of the common bile duct, with marked dilatation proximal to this involving the biliary tree'.*

Authors' Top Tip

Avoid using acronyms wherever possible. You may well get your acronyms mixed up! In all probability, the examiner will ask you to define your abbreviations anyway.

Examiner's Anecdote

'One candidate told me this was an ERPC! I asked her if she was sure, to which she replied yes! I had to explain to her that an ERPC is most definitely something very different to what this male patient had!'

Completion
- *'In summary, this patient appears to have an obstructed biliary system, secondary to gallstones.*
- *I would like to a take a focused clinical history asking specifically for symptoms suggestive of obstructive jaundice and cholecystitis, and for the older patient I would consider the possibility of a pancreatic malignancy'.*

Authors' Top Tip

When investigating this patient, you must request a serum amylase, as the patient may have gallstone pancreatitis, a diagnosis you do not want to miss!

Viva questions

Q1   What is Courvoisier's law?
In the presence of jaundice, a palpable gallbladder is unlikely to be due to stones.

(Surgical Definition)

- This means you should consider alternative diagnoses, such as cancer of the head of the pancreas.

Q2   What is Charcot's triad?
- This is a triad of abdominal pain (usually RUQ), jaundice and fever with rigors.
- It suggests the patient has ascending cholangitis, i.e. biliary sepsis.

Remember, there is a continuum of conditions that range from biliary colic to cholecystitis to finally ascending cholangitis. Patients with ascending cholangitis can deteriorate rapidly, and they usually require HDU or ITU care.

Q3   What is Calot's triangle?

(Difficult Question)

- This is the anatomical location of the cystic artery.
- It is an imaginary triangle bordered by the common hepatic duct, the cystic duct and the inferior edge of the liver.

Q4   What is Murphy's sign?
- This is the cessation of inspiration on palpation of the RUQ, which is negative on the left.
- If positive, this suggests a diagnosis of acute cholecystitis.

Case 6: Bowel Carcinoma

Instructions: This woman presented with a change in bowel habit. Comment on her film.

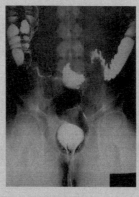

Figure 12.6: Apple core lesion

Key features to note:

- *'This is a barium follow through of Patient X, taken on Date X.*
- *The most obvious abnormality is that of a stricture in the sigmoid colon, leading to a circumferential narrowing.*
- *The margins appear shouldered, giving the characteristic apple core appearance'.*

Completion

- This patient appears to have an apple core lesion in the sigmoid colon; this strongly suggests a malignancy.
- The patient would require urgent referral to the colorectal cancer services for further management.

Most patients suspected of colon cancer have full colonoscopies; this procedure provides the advantage of being able to biopsy any lesion found during the investigation. A flexible sigmoidoscopy would reach the splenic flexure, and so may not detect more proximal tumours.

Viva Questions

Q1 How would this patient have presented?
- Left-sided tumours (as in this case) typically present with large bowel obstruction or rectal bleeding.
- However, right-sided tumours commonly present with iron deficiency anaemia due to occult blood loss (*see* Chapter 2, Case 4; and Chapter 4, Abdominal stoma examination).

Case 7: Ureteric Calculi

Instructions: This gentleman presented with loin pain. Comment on his film.

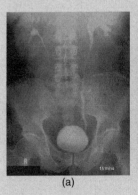 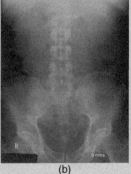

(a)	(b)

Figure 12.7: (a) IVU; (b) Control film

Key features to note:
- *'This is an intravenous urogram of Patient X, taken on Date X.*
- *It is a 15-minute contrast film; I would like to* **view the control film first***'.*

(Good Response)

Authors' Top Tip

Be careful, in the examination you may be given the contrast image first. This is not an error on the part of the examiner; he or she is testing you. Always ask to see the control film before you comment on the contrast study!

- *'On the control film, I can see two distinct opacities at the level of the left vesico-ureteric junction (VUJ); these measure X cm in size.*
- *This has led to dilatation of the proximal ureter and consequent hydronephrosis of the left kidney'.*

Completion
- *'In summary, this patient has two X-cm VUJ stones that are likely/unlikely to pass (see below).*
- *I would like to take a focused clinical history from the patient, asking specifically for left-sided colicky pain radiating to the groin, haematuria …'*

The control film is often called the X-ray KUB, which stands for kidney, ureters and bladder. This is so that when compared to a normal plain-film abdominal radiograph, the KUB film demonstrates all three major components of the renal tract, which may not always be visible on a routine film.

Traditionally, the control film is taken at time 0 minute, and the subsequent contrast films are taken at regular intervals. In theory, this can be for up to any length of time until the level of obstruction has been demonstrated or when the contrast is completely excreted by the kidneys.

The purpose of a control film is to identify any calcifications along the urinary tract from kidney to bladder that would otherwise be obscured by contrast material in the contrast film. If any calcifications are identified, then this can be compared with the contrast film to see if there is any collection of contrast material building up proximal to the lesion. This would suggest that the calcification is causing obstruction and is likely to be a stone.

It is the comparison of the two films that is crucial, as a calcification in the pelvic area of the plain-film KUB may be simply a non-specific lesion called a phlebolith, or it could be a stone impacted at the VUJ. Only by comparing the two and seeing the buildup of contrast proximal to this lesion would you diagnose this.

If a stone is identified, it is important to measure its size, as stones <4 mm in diameter are likely to pass and can be managed conservatively, whereas larger stones may need operative treatment or shockwave lithotripsy.

Most stones are composed of calcium oxalate, and as such, plain-film X-ray (KUB) will show up to 80% of all renal stones; this is in contrast to gallstones, where only 20% will be radio-opaque. Stones that occupy the entire renal pelvis are called *staghorn calculi* and need operative treatment.

Non-contrast CT KUB is now becoming the initial investigation of choice. This is mainly to exclude an AAA as a differential.

Authors' Top Tip

Be wary of the elderly patient presenting with ureteric colic; this may well be a leaking AAA. Many surgeons now say that all men >60 years of age with loin pain have a leaking AAA until proven otherwise! Keeping this in mind during your surgical on calls will do you no harm and will always prompt you to actively look for signs suggestive of an AAA.

Viva questions

Q1 What is colic?
This is the intermittent pain caused by obstruction of any hollow muscular viscus.

(Surgical Definition)

Patients with renal stones are unable to lie still due to the pain, which can be excruciating. Your first aim should be to relieve the patient's pain. An NSAID such as Diclofenac given rectally has been found to be very effective in combination with other simple analgesics. This is thought to be due to its effect in reducing ureteric peristalsis as well as its anti-inflammatory properties. Patients who need additional opiate analgesia will usually need to be admitted for pain relief.

Q2 What would you be concerned about if the patient started to spike a temperature?
- 'That there is an infection and the patient would require antibiotics'.

(Good Response)

- *'That the patient has an infected and obstructed system which will require intravenous antibiotics and urgent surgical management in the form of a percutaneous nephrostomy to decompress the system.*
- *This is to prevent renal failure and septicaemia, which can be life-threatening'.*

(Honours Response)

Q3 Can a patient with ureteric colic be sent home from the emergency department?

(Difficult Question)

Say that you would first discuss with a urologist, but generally patients can be discharged if:
- The stone is likely to pass (i.e. it is in the distal third of the ureter and is <4 mm).
- There are no signs of coexisting infection, i.e. the patient is apyrexial and has a minimally raised white cell count.

- There is normal renal function (i.e. minimal hydronephrosis on CT).
- The patient has minimal pain that is adequately managed with simple analgesia.

Patients are also usually sent home with Tamsulosin, an alpha-1 blocker. The distal ureter contains alpha-adrenoceptors therefore Tamsulosin aids in the expulsion of small distal ureteric stones and reduces the frequency of ureteric colic.

Q4 What are the various anatomical points in the urinary tract where stones can lodge?

(Difficult Question)

- There are several sites of narrowing in the urinary tract, including the pelvi-ureteric junction (PUJ), at the pelvic brim where the iliac vessels cross the vesico-ureteric junction (VUJ).

(Good Response)

- Renal calculi tend to cause luminal obstruction at various anatomically narrow points throughout the course of the ureters.
- The kidneys lie obliquely along the psoas muscle with their upper poles at the level of T12.
- The first anatomical point of narrowing is at the junction where the pelvis joins the ureter, the PUJ.
- The ureter then leaves the hilum and courses along just lateral to the tips of the transverse vertebral processes, where it crosses the pelvic brim at the sacroiliac joint, which is the second site of anatomical narrowing.
- The ureter then continues towards the ischial spine but curves medially towards the base of the bladder where it enters obliquely at the last point of anatomical narrowing, the VUJ.

(Honours Response)

Case 8: Large bowel obstruction

Instructions: This woman presented with abdominal pain. Comment on her film.

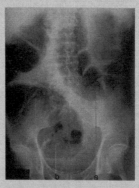

Figure 12.8: Bowel obstruction

Key features to note:

- *'This is a plain-film abdominal radiograph of Patient X, taken on Date X.*
- *The most obvious abnormality is that of multiple, dilated loops of bowel.* [Offer to measure the diameter in centimetres.]
- *These are peripherally placed, with visible haustra* (a)*, and so they are most likely to be large bowel'.*

(Good Response)

- *'The caecum is also markedly dilated* (b)*, indicating that the ileo-caecal valve is competent'.*

(Honours Response)

Authors' Top Tip

A markedly dilated caecum in a patient with bowel obstruction indicates a competent ileo-caecal valve. If you purposefully look for this whenever you review a film suggestive of bowel obstruction, you are demonstrating to the examiner that you are actively looking for the associated complications of bowel obstruction and thereby demonstrating your breadth of knowledge. Bowel obstruction in the presence of a competent ileo-caecal valve is called a closed-loop obstruction. The competent valve essentially prevents air from escaping into the small bowel proximally and consequently accelerates the distension of large bowel and increases the risk of perforation.

Completion

- *'In summary, this patient has large bowel obstruction. As the patient appears to have a competent ileo-caecal valve, I am concerned about the high risk for perforation'.*

In bowel obstruction, look for diameters of >5 cm; the critical diameter before perforation is likely is 9 cm, and >12 cm indicates imminent perforation; therefore, it is essential to measure the diameter.

In some cases, the AXR may even demonstrate the cause of bowel obstruction due to, e.g. a sigmoid volvulus:

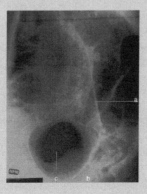

Figure 12.9: Sigmoid volvulus a: Coffee bean sign, b: Convergence point c: Grossly distended sigmoid

When a bowel segment twists through 360°, this compromises its circulation, leaving it susceptible to gangrene and perforation. This is called a volvulus. A sigmoid volvulus can be managed conservatively with endoscopic decompression using a flatus tube, which is inserted through a rigid sigmoidoscope. If the volvulus cannot be untwisted, then the patient will need operative treatment.

Viva questions

Q1 What are the causes of bowel obstruction?
- In general, the most common causes of bowel obstruction in this country are postoperative adhesions, followed by hernias and cancers.
- Small bowel obstruction is more common than large bowel.
- The most common causes of small bowel obstruction are adhesions, hernias and cancers.
- The most common causes for large bowel obstruction are cancer, diverticular disease or a volvulus.

(Good Response)

- Although there are many causes of bowel obstruction, they can generally be divided into mechanical and non-mechanical causes.
- Mechanical causes can be classified according to their relation to the bowel wall, as in the lumen (luminal), in the wall, or outside the wall (extramural):

Table 12.4: Mechanical causes

Location	Pathology
Luminal	Gallstones, meconium, intussusception, impacted faeces, worms, foreign bodies, etc.
Extramural	Adhesions, cancers, hernias, volvulus.
In the wall	Congenital stenosis, strictures, inflammatory bowel disease, diverticulitis, cancer, radiation colitis.

- A non-mechanical cause, also known as a paralytic ileus, is commonly due to postoperative abdominal surgery (which is prolonged beyond the normal duration of bowel inactivity), mesenteric ischaemia, peritonitis and from metabolic causes such as hypokalaemia, uraemia, hyperglycaemia and hypothyroidism. It can also occur due to the side effects of anticholinergic drugs.
- Another type of functional bowel obstruction is a phenomenon called pseudo-obstruction, where the bowel appears to be affected by mechanical obstruction but there is no mechanical cause found. This is managed conservatively.

(Honours Response)

Authors' Top Tip

The average student responds to this question by stating the most common causes. While this is correct, it is an insufficient answer. The top students are able to demonstrate their breath of knowledge by answering using a classic anatomical sieve as a framework in which to deliver their answers.

Q2   How do you know this is large bowel and not small bowel obstruction, radiologically?

Table 12.5: Small versus large bowel

Bowel	Radiological features
Small	Valvulae conniventes (mucosal folds across the entire bowel lumen), central position of bowel.
Large	Incomplete haustral folds, peripheral position of bowel, markedly distended caecum.

Q3   What are the cardinal features of bowel obstruction in a history?
- Central, colicky abdominal pain.
- Vomiting.
- Absolute constipation, i.e. no flatus or faeces.
- Abdominal distension.

Q4   How can you differentiate between small and large bowel obstruction from the history?

(Difficult Question)

Table 12.6: History of obstruction

History	Small bowel	Large bowel
Pain	Central abdominal pain	Central and lower abdominal pain
Vomiting	Occurs early	Late feature with strangulation
Constipation	Occurs late	Occurs early
Distension	Less distension	More distension

Q5   How would you manage this patient?
- The patient would need to be started on intravenous fluids and given a nasogastric tube for decompression.

(Average Response)

Authors' Top Tip

Questions asking about management involve taking a focused history and clinical examination, as well as discussing the actual treatment options. So make sure you put this across in your answer. Remember, whenever investigating the acute abdomen, you must always rule out pancreatitis and an AAA.

- 'This is a surgical emergency. I would resuscitate the patient, ensuring his or her airway is patent, breathing is adequate and address the patient's circulation by inserting two large-bore cannulae whilst taking blood for further investigation at the same time'. (*see* below)
- 'I will then begin the patient on aggressive fluid resuscitation, as the patient is likely to have suffered significant third-space loss'. [Large volumes of fluid can sequester in the bowel.]

Investigations

- **Bloods:** FBC, U&E, serum amylase, G&S; ABG in more unwell patients.
- **X-rays:** Erect CXR looking for free air under the diaphragm, indicating perforated bowel (*see* Case 4); AXR looking for obstruction.
- **Enema:** A water-soluble contrast can be injected per rectum in cases of mechanical bowel obstruction to assess for free flow around the bowel. This can even be therapeutic.
- **CT abdomen:** This can determine the level of obstruction, identify the cause and check bowel viability.

Treatment

Conservative measures include:
- Keeping the patient NBM.
- Inserting a nasogastric tube for decompression and IV fluids; this is the so-called 'drip and suck' regimen.
- Analgesia and supplemental oxygen.

Regarding surgical measures:
- These should be considered if conservative treatment has failed after 48 hrs, or there are signs of strangulation.
- Some patients may undergo colonic stenting, otherwise the aims of surgery are to decompress the bowel and resect any non-viable bowel.
- In some cases, patients may have an emergency Hartmann's procedure (*see* Chapter 2, Case 4; and Chapter 4, Abdominal stoma examination).

Q6 Would you give a barium enema to a patient with mechanical bowel obstruction?

(Difficult Question)

- No, barium is peritonitic; if you give this and there is in fact a perforation, you have just given the patient peritonitis and made things worse!
- You should use a water-soluble contrast material such as gastrograffin, as it is diagnostic and in some cases therapeutic, e.g. it relieves some of the adhesional obstructions.

Q7 Do you know of any laws that govern the pressure inside the bowel?

(Honours Question)

- Laplace's law states that as pressure increases, the tension in a tubular wall is maximal at the point where the diameter of the tube is at its greatest.

- For bowel obstruction, the important structure to keep in mind is the caecum. This is because it has the greatest diameter and the thinnest wall. Therefore, the caecum is the site most likely to perforate first.

Case 9: Post-traumatic abdomen   (Honours Case)

Instructions: This man was involved in an RTA. Comment on his scan.

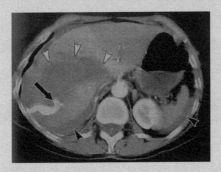

Figure 12.10: CT liver laceration

Key features to note:
- *'This is a CT abdomen of Patient X, taken Date X; this is a single slice.*
- *The most obvious abnormality is that of multiple low-attenuation areas of varying size in the liver* [white arrow heads].
- *There are further areas of low attenuation around the spleen and the liver edge posteriorly* [black arrow heads].
- *This free fluid in the abdomen is most likely to be blood.*
- *I can also see an area of high attenuation over the lateral aspect of the liver posteriorly* [black arrow], *this appears to be contrast material that is acutely extravasating from a large liver laceration'.*

<u>**Completion**</u>
- *'In summary, this patient has a large liver laceration leading to active bleeding.*
- *This is a surgical emergency, and the patient should be managed according to ATLS principles.*
- *It is likely, however, that the patient will require urgent surgical intervention to control the bleeding'.*

Authors' Top Tip

When students see this image, they often panic. Do not be afraid of a CT scan; the pathology is usually obvious. Even if you are stuck, you may ask the examiner for more history to help you. The examiner is not testing your ability to read CT scans; he or she will most likely expect you to discuss the management of this patient from an ATLS perspective. The actual pathology on the scan is irrelevant.

Case 10: Oesophageal rupture   (Honours Case)

Instructions: This man presented with chest pain. Comment on his film.

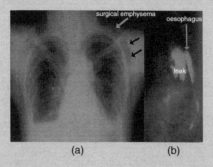

(a)   (b)

Figure 12.11: Oesophageal perforation a: CXR, b: Contrast swallow

Key features to note:
- *'This is a chest radiograph of Patient X, taken on Date X.*
- *The most obvious abnormality is that of air in the subcutaneous tissues (surgical emphysema) and mediastinum.*
- *There is an associated pleural effusion on the right and an area of consolidation on the left.*
- *The contrast swallow demonstrates a leak in the oesophagus, which is the likely cause of the CXR findings'.*

Completion
- *'In summary, my findings are consistent with a diagnosis of oesophageal perforation.*
- *This is a surgical emergency ...'*

We hope this case demonstrates to you what we expect an honours case to entail. You are expected to not only report a film but also think and actively look for causes of what you find. The second image of a contrast swallow was only provided if you specifically asked for it. By requesting a contrast swallow, you are demonstrating the level required to be awarded an honours mark, as you are actively thinking about what you would do next in actual clinical practice.

This particular case was due to spontaneous rupture of the oesophagus, but the most common cause of oesophageal perforation is iatrogenic, i.e. an endoscopy causing instrumental perforation. This is because there are several sites along the oesophagus where it is prone to rupture due to anatomical narrowing (*see* Chapter 2, Case 6: Viva Q4).

And so, when investigating such a patient, a water-soluble contrast such as Visipaque is essential, as barium leaking can lead to life-threatening mediastinitis. There may be air in the mediastinum or soft tissues on CXR with a consequent pleural effusion. Classically, when auscultating the heart you will hear a mediastinal crunch. The mainstay of treatment involves keeping the patient NBM, starting IV antibiotics and inserting a chest drain. Specific surgical management involves repairing the perforation via a thoracotomy.

Index

Tables and diagrams are given in italics